CRITICAL DECISIONS

Also by Peter Ubel
  Pricing Life
  You're Stronger than You Think
  Free Market Madness

CRITICAL DECISIONS

*How You and Your Doctor
Can Make the Right Medical
Choices Together*

PETER A. UBEL, M.D.

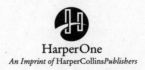

HarperOne
An Imprint of HarperCollinsPublishers

For Paula

HarperOne

CRITICAL DECISIONS: *How You and Your Doctor Can Make the Right Medical Decisions Together.* Copyright © 2012 by Peter A. Ubel. All rights reserved. Printed in the United States of America. No part of this book may be used or reproduced in any manner whatsoever without written permission except in the case of brief quotations embodied in critical articles and reviews. For information, address HarperCollins Publishers, 10 East 53rd Street, New York, NY 10022.

HarperCollins books may be purchased for educational, business, or sales promotional use. For information, please e-mail the Special Markets Department at SPsales@harpercollins.com.

HarperCollins website: http://www.harpercollins.com

HarperCollins®, ⛃®, and HarperOne™ are
trademarks of HarperCollins Publishers

Designed by Level C

FIRST EDITION

Library of Congress Cataloging-in-Publication Data
Ubel, Peter A.
Critical decisions : how you and your doctor can make the right medical choices together /
Peter A. Ubel.—1st ed.
p. cm.
ISBN 978-0-06-210382-6
1. Medicine—Decision making. 2. Clinical medicine—Decision making. 3. Physician and patient. 4. Choice (Psychology) I. Title.
R723.5.U24 2012
610.69'6—dc23
2012007934

12 13 14 15 16 RRD(H) 10 9 8 7 6 5 4 3 2 1

CONTENTS

PROLOGUE
Who's in Charge?

In the old days, Fred Furelli wouldn't have been allowed to feel so miserably unsure of his decision. His doctor would have made the decision for him. But now he lay in bed at night worried and bewildered. The urologist had told him he had early-stage prostate cancer, and the tumor could be cured with either surgery or radiation, or—and this was hard to fathom—he could do nothing, wait to see if the cancer grows.

He contemplated his options. The urologist had laid out a slew of information on what surgery would feel like, but in the aftermath of learning he had cancer, that information was a blur. The urologist had not discussed radiation as thoroughly as surgery. Was this a sign that it wasn't a viable option? As for the third option, he was still perplexed that a cancer could be bad enough to warrant an operation yet mild enough to address with "watchful waiting." Things weren't adding up.

So he came to me for advice.

I was Mr. Furelli's primary care internist, and we had known each other for half a decade. (Like all the patients in this book, Furelli's name is a pseudonym.) I had seen his pathology report as well as his urologist's assessment of his condition. His cancer was small and hadn't traveled beyond the prostate gland. Furelli was in his early seventies, which meant there was a decent chance his tiny cancer would smolder for years without affecting his health. Hence the option of watchful waiting. With this approach, the urologist would test his blood at regular intervals to see if his cancer was growing fast enough to threaten his health, at which point we would reconsider the risks and benefits of more aggressive approaches.

But not everyone is comfortable waiting around while an alien-like presence grows inside him. Watchful waiting feels too passive for some men. (Some urologists have even renamed this approach "active surveillance" to overcome this perception.) More aggressive treatments, however—such as surgery and radiation—are not benign little procedures. The vast majority of men receiving these treatments experience impotence and urinary incontinence. In other words, patients recover from these arduous treatments only to discover that they have trouble with erections and need to wear adult diapers.

My patient was completely torn. He didn't like the idea of going through a painful treatment, nor of suffering from treatment complications. But he wasn't crazy about doing "nothing" either, as he put it to me. That's the reason he asked for my advice.

It's also the reason I wrote this book, to lay out the dilemma I faced that day: whether I should give him advice or leave him to make up his own mind. I took care of Mr. Furelli in the mid- to late 1990s, two decades into the patient-empowerment revolution. Prior to the revolution, medical decisions weren't shared affairs. Doctors made decisions and patients largely obeyed. Indeed, physicians had dominated medical decision making for the better part of two millennia, from the time of Hippocrates through the dawn of medical science in the twentieth century straight up until the mid-1970s, when the traditions of medical decision making ran head-on into patients (and lawyers and a new breed of people called ethicists) who demanded that doctors involve patients more actively in their decisions.

I was quite aware of the revolution as I cared for Mr. Furelli. At the time, you see, I was an assistant professor of medicine at the University of Pennsylvania and one of the founding faculty members of that school's Center for Bioethics. A philosophy major as an undergrad, I had studied bioethics at the University of Chicago after completing my medical training. I'm not spouting off my CV to impress you but to explain where I was coming from on that day. I was a new breed of physician. Swept up by the moral momentum of the revolution, I was determined to be the kind of doctor who didn't boss around his patients. I wouldn't tell patients what to do; I'd help patients make their own decisions.

In the prerevolutionary days of physician paternalism, this patient's urologist would have told him that he had a small growth in his prostate and needed surgery. Or, if the surgeon felt that the patient was too frail to benefit from surgery, he would have withheld information about the tumor and monitored it without the patient's knowledge. As the word *paternalism* suggests, the old days were modeled on parent–child relationships, with the doctor acting as the all-powerful and knowing parent, benevolently protecting the childlike patient from worry and responsibility. If the patient were deemed too fragile for bad news, the doctor would turn to euphemism or out-and-out evasion. The tumor would be described as "an X-ray shadow" or "an infection." In those days, doctors made the decisions and patients were expected to follow their orders.

Back then, this gentleman would not have lain awake at night wondering what to do. But today Mr. Furelli was torn asunder by indecision and came to me looking for help.

"What would you do if you had this cancer?" he asked me.

New Age doctor that I was, I threw him back into his pool of indecision. "This is your decision to make."

He looked confused.

"Let me try an example," I said. "What are you going to watch on TV tonight?"

"The hockey game," he responded, an altogether unsurprising response given the Philadelphia Flyers hat perched on his balding head.

"Bad decision," I shot back. "You should watch the figure-skating competition on channel 19 instead."

He looked at me incredulously. "But I don't like figure skating."

"Exactly!" I exclaimed. "I can't tell you what to watch on TV tonight because the 'right' choice depends on your preferences. The same thing goes for your prostate cancer."

My bioethics training had taught me that the best choice is often not merely a *medical* decision but instead hinges on a patient's values. The best choice for this patient, in fact, depended on how important he felt it was to avoid treatment complications, such as urinary incontinence, versus how he felt about the prospect of living with an untreated cancer. Steeped in bioethical theories, I had brilliantly taught this patient the difference between facts and values, the distinction between medical judgments and patients' rights.

Mr. Furelli seemed to understand my point. He looked at me with a knowing glance and said, "Okay, Doc. What would you do if you were me?"

My brilliant analogy hadn't empowered him as much as I had expected.

I SHOULD HAVE KNOWN BETTER

I should have known better than to foist this decision upon my reluctant patient. By that time I had been practicing medicine for about a decade, and I'd had hundreds of patients ask me for my medical advice: "What should I do, Doc?" or "What would you do if it were your mother, Doctor?" These requests, and a dozen similar variations, had become daily invitations for me to impart my supposed wisdom upon grateful patients, wisdom that was not limited to medical knowledge. I didn't just help people figure out which pill would control their blood pressure with the fewest side effects. I was helping men figure out how to tell their spouses they'd caught herpes. I found myself imparting marital advice before I was married, childrearing tips before I'd had children, and end-of-life guidance before any of my close friends or relatives had died.

I'd come to learn that patients don't want their doctors to simply toss medical information at them and let them figure out what to do. So I should have known better than to believe a figure-skating analogy would suddenly empower my patient to become an independent decision maker. Rightly or wrongly, many patients value their doctor's advice and indeed rely on such advice when they are overwhelmed by the situation at hand. I expect many readers would react the same as Furelli, looking for guidance and advice in a time of need, not seeking to establish decision-making authority. In turning the decision back on Mr. Furelli with my skating analogy, I'd come face-to-face with the myth of patient empowerment. Mr. Furelli had been educated about his treatment alternatives and about the importance of his values in making the right decision, but all this information and freedom of choice didn't leave him feeling very empowered. Leaders of the patient-empowerment revolution had fought a battle in favor of patient autonomy over physician paternalism. Disgusted by the way physicians dominated medical decision making, they had worked to make patients into the decision makers, thereby relegating physicians to the role of information providers. Jerome Groopman espoused this view in an interview on *The Colbert Report*. In his inimitable manner, Colbert had asked Groopman who really ought to make medical decisions: "Are you saying that I get to decide on my treatment? Why did you go to medical school?" Groopman responded to Colbert much the way I had tried to respond to Mr. Furelli that day: "I went to medical school to help you understand the risks and benefits as an individual, so you can put your values into the decision."

Information and integration—that's what some physicians see as the new paradigm. Leaders of the revolution had believed that the problem with medical care was that patients had no power, and they saw information as the cure. But most patients don't want their doctors to act merely as information providers. They don't want their doctors to deflect requests for guidance with awkward figure-skating analogies or appeals to "put your values into the decision."

So what's a better alternative? Carl Schneider, a lawyer and bioethics expert at the University of Michigan, has written that if we really want to respect patient "autonomy," if we want to let patients have more say over their medical decisions, then we need to respect their right to let the doctor make the decision.

Yet I was hesitant to give Mr. Furelli the recommendation he wanted, not because I thought he had a duty to make the decision but because I worried that his desire to defer to me was less a reflection of his decision-making preferences than it was a result of unconscious forces influencing his stated desires. I felt that way, in large part, because during my ethics training I had wandered over from the philosophy department to the behavioral sciences building and collaborated with behavioral economists and decision psychologists, from whom I learned about the emotional and irrational influences that shape people's decisions, influences that often cause people to back off from difficult decisions.

Take a classic decision-making study led by Amos Tversky and Eldar Shafir. The two psychologists asked Princeton undergrads to imagine themselves walking to the library to study one night and, along the way, noticing a poster for a foreign film they had always wanted to see. The undergrads were then asked whether they would continue on to the library or go to the film. Only 20 percent of Princeton students said they would continue on to the library. The point of this study, however, was not to see whether Princeton undergrads were studious; Tversky and Shafir wanted to discover what would happen when the students faced a slightly more complicated choice. They then presented half of the students with a different scenario, asking them to imagine walking to the library to study and this time seeing not only a poster for a foreign film but also an announcement for what looked like a fascinating lecture. Whatever you think about the idea of attending a "fascinating lecture," you'll have to agree that, with more alternatives available, even fewer students should choose to go to the library. But that's not what Tversky and Shafir discovered. Instead, they found that a whopping 40 percent of students said they would go to the library.

The moral of this study is that when decisions get even a little tough, many people look for ways not to decide. Now imagine my patient, Mr. Furelli, who was facing a much more complicated and consequential decision. Is it any wonder that he wanted a way to avoid the decision? And what better way than to ask his doctor to make the decision for him? Illness often forces people to face incredibly complex and emotionally frightening choices. It is only natural for patients in such cases to look to their physicians for advice. That's why even at the beginning of my career, when I must have looked like Doogie Howser, M.D. (I barely needed to shave and looked much younger than my advanced age of twenty-six), I found octogenarians asking me for advice on life-and-death decisions.

That's why, when Mr. Furelli asked for my help in deciding about his prostate cancer, I should have known better than to think that a thirty-second primer on autonomy would overcome his indecision. My figure-skating trick was naïve. An honest mistake, I thought at the time, a noble failure. I was trying to empower this patient so that his preferences would dictate his treatment course.

I'll return to Mr. Furelli's decision much later in this book, and show how his story illustrates an alternative to the dichotomous choice between patient autonomy and physician paternalism, but first we need to look more closely at this whole idea that patient preferences ought to drive medical decisions.

WHAT DOES "BETTER" MEAN?

"Preferences" is a key word in current debates about freedom and well-being. If people have stable preferences—things that represent their individual view of "the good life"—and if these preferences vary from one person to another (I like tomatoes, you like tomahtos?), then the right choice will also vary from person to person. In such situations a one-size-fits-all policy will harm people. Better instead to give people freedom to decide, one at a time, what they prefer.

Chalk that up as another thing I should have known better than to believe, because a wealth of scientific evidence has shown that people often don't have strong preferences. Many people's preferences instead vacillate from one moment to the next. I know this from my own research, much of which explores the unconscious and irrational forces that influence medical decisions, causing people's decision-making "preferences" to shift with subtle changes in how treatments are described.

For instance, people are much more inclined to opt for a surgical procedure with a 90 percent survival rate than one with a 10 percent mortality rate, even though that's simply two different ways of describing the same surgery. It's not just that people get confused about the math. Instead, these two ways of framing the decision *feel* different. I'll explore some of the reasons for such feelings later. For now, though, let it suffice that on the day I presented the figure-skating analogy to my anxious patient, I should have known better than to think that my moral duty was to force him to make this decision himself. The moral importance of getting patients to make choices diminishes as patient choices become more arbitrary and less tied to what patients value.

There's one more reason I should have been a better doctor that day. I had already had enough experience as a patient to know that patient autonomy is not everything ethicists have touted it as being. Take, for example, my first orthopedic operation:

I was twenty-nine years old when a sudden change of direction on a softball field caused a pain to shoot down my right leg. I had squashed my fourth lumbar disc (the disc between L4 and L5, to be precise), leaving it nowhere to go but into the space reserved for the nerve supplying my right leg.

After a round of physical therapy and rest, I met with a surgeon who said he could remove the protruding part of my disc, but it would require a fairly big operation. (These days, such surgeries are typically less invasive.) Alternatively, my surgeon said, I could give the injury more time to heal and see if the disc shrank enough that I could resume athletic activities.

At the time of this injury, I was a medical resident at the Mayo Clinic, and during my training I'd become quite familiar with the hospital library. When I saw a patient in the hospital, I would run to the library to read up on their problems. If one of my patients had a rare infection, I'd scour the literature for the best antibiotic. If a patient presented with an unusual constellation of symptoms, I'd dig around in books, looking for a unifying diagnosis.

So you can only imagine the literature scouring I performed when my own health was under threat. Hours in the library? Days, maybe? Try: I never got around to it. I never researched my own health condition. Instead, like a powerless child, I looked to Papa Surgeon for advice. He suggested I get the operation. I also spoke with my residency director and asked him what he thought I should do.

All the while, the obvious course of action was staring me in the face. With physical therapy, I had discovered I could tolerate the pain pretty well. I could bike and swim. And with enough time, if the disc continued to shrink and abandon its home on the side of my nerve root, I'd be able to resume most of my other activities.

Not that hard of a decision, really. Take time and see what happens. But there was one complicating factor. My residency ended in two months, at which point I was moving to the University of Chicago. I spoke to my residency director about my fears, and he told me, "You're at the Mayo Clinic now, Peter, with the best surgeons in the world. You might not need the operation today, but do you really want to move to Chicago worried that you are one fart away from emergency surgery?"

He was kidding about the fart, of course. A tiny puff of wind wouldn't push the disc further toward my nerve root. Nevertheless, that image hit me at my brain stem, "One fart," I thought, "and I might need emergency surgery!"

So here I was, Mr. Rational, a philosophy major who prided himself on logic and reasoning, a newly trained physician who practiced evidence-based medicine. And instead of letting the medical literature guide my decision (literature that would have screamed at me to wait), I was persuaded to undergo spinal surgery because of a fart joke.

Why would I think, half a dozen years later, that a figure-skating analogy would turn a scared seventy-two-year-old man into a decision-making expert?

ALL INFORMED AND NOWHERE TO GO

In the first part of this book, I tell the story of the patient-empowerment revolution—how over a handful of tumultuous years in the mid-1970s medical practice was transformed from a two-thousand-year-old tradition of "doctor knows best" to a brave new world of patients' rights. In the second part, I paint a picture of how this revolution has worked out for doctors and patients. It ain't always a pretty picture. I tell stories of doctors and patients stumbling through difficult decisions—unaware of how they're being influenced by emotions, cognitive illusions, even fart jokes—with discussion of the science that illuminates their decision processes. I also dig into the nitty-gritty of how doctors and patients talk with each other as they confront these decisions. I'm sad to say that these conversations often reveal a canyon-size gulf between doctors and patients, one that shows patient empowerment to be an impossible ideal.

Consider Jim Leech, a man who let me tape-record a conversation he had with his urologist. Leech had been waiting almost a week for the result of his prostate biopsy. He had peed blood for several days and had taken pain pills until he got sick of feeling drowsy. When the moment of truth arrived, he sat in front of the urologist, waiting to hear what the biopsy revealed. His urologist chatted with him about his recovery from the biopsy and then gave him the bad news.

"So we took twelve cores out of your prostate," the urologist began. "Out of those there were three cores that had cancer in them, and the percentage of the cores that was cancer was fairly low. It was under 30 percent. So out of those three cores—that are about, you know, this long—a third of them had a little bit of cancer in them. So those three cores out of twelve says that there's probably not an extensive amount of prostate cancer in your prostate. But we should talk about different treatment options."

The urologist continued, without interruption. If you didn't catch what he said, he'd just told Leech that he had prostate cancer.

"We also grade prostate cancer on how it looks under the microscope. We give it a score between 6 and 10."

"Is that the Teason?" Mr. Leech asked.

"That's the Gleason score."

"Oh, Gleason score. Okay," the patient replied.

"Yep, so 6 is what we consider the most low-grade, least aggressive-looking, but it's the most . . . it's just abnormal enough for us to call it cancer. If it were any less than that, if there were less atypical-looking cells, we couldn't call it cancer. So it's just enough to get a grade of cancer and then that goes all the way up to a score of 10, which is very abnormal looking and is more aggressive."

"But 6 is the beginning number?"

"Yes, 6 is the least aggressive, 10 is the most aggressive."

"I'm used to, like, 1," Leech said, laughing.

"Yeah, well, the way we typically split it up is into thirds—low risk, intermediate risk, and high risk."

"Right."

"Low risk is Gleason 6, intermediate is usually 7s—either 3+4 or 4+3, depending on how it looks under the microscope—and then 8, 9, and 10 are all high risk. So yours was an intermediate risk. So it's in the middle. It was 3+3 and 3+4, so just enough of the atypical cells of the grade 4 to make it 3+4, which means you're intermediate risk."

In the old days of physician paternalism, remember, doctors didn't tell patients when they had cancer, out of concern that patients couldn't handle the news. But now that physicians have moved on to the new paradigm, patients like Leech not only learn that they have cancer but also receive soliloquies filled with enough technical details to satisfy the most rigorously peer-reviewed medical journal. Taught that their patients deserve information about their conditions, physicians don't know how far their pedagogical duties extend. Consequently, their patients are often left wallowing in a swamp of irrelevant information. Does it matter that this person's "7" was a 3+4 rather than a 4+3? And does anyone think that, mere seconds after learning that he has cancer, this man is ready to absorb this kind of arcane information?

Jim Leech was one of a few hundred men who participated in a study I conducted with Angie Fagerlin, a psychologist at the University of Michigan who studies decision making. Early in this study, we transcribed audiotapes of a half-dozen encounters, including Leech's, and convened a conference call of the research team to discuss ways of analyzing these conversations. At one point I suggested that we evaluate what urologists were doing to help people emotionally absorb the bad news, pointing out that in cases like Mr. Leech's, the urologist had rapidly segued from delivering the bad news ("there were three cores that had cancer in them") to technical discussions of tumor grade ("we give it a score between 6 and 10"), without any time for emotional reflection.

My suggestion put one of the urologists on the defensive. "It's not like they're getting bad news," she said.

Huh? Finding out you have cancer isn't bad news?

The urologist was speaking from the perspective of a clinical expert who knew that localized prostate cancer is a very treatable disease, who knew that most of these patients would not die of this cancer, who was deeply aware of just how well most men cope with this illness. But the urologist didn't have a clue about what Jim Leech would feel when he heard the news. "Isn't it possible," I gently replied, "that patients will *feel* like this diagnosis is bad news?"

My question was met with incredulity. So we moved on to other topics.

Later in our conversation, I pointed out that the urologists we had tape-recorded appeared to be overwhelming patients with information. My urologist collaborator shot back, "Well, it's not like the patients are having a hard time understanding the information."

"How do you know that?" I asked.

"They aren't asking any questions," the urologist replied.

When doctors ruled, standing tall on their paternalistic pedestals, they didn't worry about whether their patients understood their medical situations. All they cared about was making sure that their patients did what they, the doctors, thought the patients ought to do: take this pill, stay in bed for this many days, take an aspirin and call me in the morning. Knocked off this pedestal, doctors no longer know where to stand. They're trying to find a balance between giving too much information to patients and too little, between telling patients what to do and leaving them to their own devices.

Keep this conversation about prostate cancer not being "bad news" in mind the next time you see a doctor, as a reminder that the way you feel during the appointment may not be apparent to your physician. A bit of news might scare you or an explanation may leave you confused, but if you don't explicitly discuss your fear or your confusion, your doctor will probably assume everything is hunky-dory.

One of my goals in writing this book is to help patients and future patients (and aren't we all future patients?) to recognize what's going on in their doctors' minds when they interact. As will become clear, too often doctors don't grasp what's going on in their patients' minds, and patients return the favor by failing to recognize what's going on in their doctors' minds. Leech's urologist was probably convinced that Leech was soothed by the thorough description of his tumor staging that he had described. (He probably figured anyone would be relieved to learn that his cancer was only a Gleason 7, and a 3+4 one at that.) Leech might have concluded that his urologist was an uncaring technocrat, more interested in tumor pathology than his patient's feelings. My guess is that Leech's urologist cared deeply about his patient's emotions but didn't have enough of a grasp on what Leech was feeling to communicate accordingly. On both ends of the stethoscope, two people whose backgrounds and experiences conspired against their attempts to understand each other.

DIFFICULT ADVICE TO SWALLOW

William Engmann was admitted to my hospital service in the winter of 2007 because he could no longer swallow. This inability to swallow, what we doctors call dysphagia, was his only medical complaint, one that snuck up on him over the course of a month. For some unknown reason, he couldn't find the muscular strength to propel food and liquid down to his stomach.

After running tests, we discovered that Engmann had metastatic lung cancer, his tumor having spread beyond the confines of his lung. In response, his immune system was counterattacking, producing antibodies and white blood cells designed to thwart the cancer. But these defense mechanisms were causing collateral damage. To his immune system, the tumor cells looked a lot like his throat muscles, so it had started attacking those cells too. That's why he couldn't swallow.

Engmann's cancer was incurable. But we nevertheless wanted to treat him, in the hopes of slowing down the progression of his tumor, so he'd have a few extra months of life and perhaps even a chance to swallow again before he died.

This man's situation was tragic. In his mid-fifties, with a loving wife and several children ready to start families of their own, he was understandably distressed about his situation. We had arranged for him to have a feeding tube, and I came by to see him the morning after the tube was placed to see how he was doing. I checked his abdomen for signs of infection and, more importantly, assessed his fragile mood. I made small talk while examining his belly and something about his response and the look he gave his wife told me things weren't right. I asked him how he was feeling, keeping purposely vague about whether I was posing a medical or social question. His wife responded forcefully, lashing out at her husband for having snuck off that morning to grab a smoke. He glared back at her, with the kind of evil-eyes-of-death look that only a spouse can give, and told her to "mind her own business."

She looked toward me for support. I was the antitobacco medical doctor, after all. But I found myself in a tough position. Was it my duty to tell this patient what to do? Or should I simply give him the information about the risks and benefits of smoking, à la Groopman, and let him make up his own mind?

According to the new ethical paradigm of preference-sensitive decision making, doctors shouldn't tell patients what to do. Rather, we should educate our patients about the risks and benefits of their options. But despite this new paradigm, I couldn't sit back that day and merely inform this man about the pros and cons of tobacco. I couldn't stand by in the role of a dispassionate educator and let him hurt himself. Instead, I felt compelled to give him advice that would promote his best interests.

I told him to smoke.

"You two obviously love each other very much," I said. "I know that you [looking at his wife] are trying to keep your husband from smoking because you love him and don't want him to get sicker. But those cigarettes aren't going to hurt him now. If anything, they'll help him relax. What matters is that you two stick together, because these next few months are going to be really difficult."

I reminded Engmann and his wife that his cancer wasn't curable and that we were mainly hoping to improve his quality of life, not to provide him a way out of his death sentence. And I explained that the best way to maximize the quality of his remaining life was to spend quality time with the people he loved. Arguing with his wife was not going to make things better.

I'm telling this story now for a couple of reasons. First, this story captures part of my evolution as a physician and scholar writing about shared decision making. By the time I took care of Engmann, I no longer believed my decision-making duty was limited to being that of an information provider. I had come to believe that shared decision making required more back-and-forth between my patients and me. I had learned that being a physician gave me a different perspective on how illness affects people's lives, and I had come to believe that it is a dereliction of my duty to withhold my perspective from patients when I can improve their lives by sharing my perspective.

Sometimes that means encouraging my patients to smoke.

But was I right to be so assertive? When, if ever, is such assertiveness proper and when is it simply a power grab? And how did we, as a society, end up in a place where doctors like me, and their patients too, find themselves unsure about who is supposed to be deciding what?

The second reason I am telling you this story is to raise these who-should-be-deciding-what questions. The patient-empowerment revolution has left many doctors and patients struggling to figure out their proper role in medical decision making. The revolution created a shift in the relationship between doctors and patients, in determining who has final authority over medical decisions. But the revolution hasn't worked out the way most of us had hoped. Too often it has left doctors and patients caught between paradigms. "Should I urge this patient to undergo treatment?" the physician wonders. "Is it a cop-out if I ask my doctor for advice?" the patient asks.

In the third and fourth parts of this book, I point the way toward a more balanced paradigm, one that doesn't pit doctors and patients against each other but instead pulls them together to make decisions, with each party giving what they are best suited to contribute to the decision. The scientific understanding of decision making, and of doctor–patient communication, has advanced enough in the previous few decades that we are ready to bring patients and doctors together from across the divide. It starts with helping each party understand what the other person is thinking. In part III, I tell the story of shared decision-making advocates who've developed "decision aids" to better inform patients about their medical alternatives, without relying on doctors to do all the dirty work. Recognizing that doctors aren't always up to the task of educating patients about their health conditions ("it was 3+3 and 3+4"), they've built a library of booklets, DVDs, and websites that patients can comb over in preparation for their doctor appointments. I show the promise of such materials. I even provide tips to all of you future patients, about how you can get more involved in your medical decisions in order to make better choices or communicate more effectively with your doctor so that he or she will give you better advice.

The new revolution in medical care needs to be less about power and more about partnership. The best decisions are often shared ones.

And there should be no silent partners in medical decision making. At a minimum, we need to prepare patients to communicate their preferences more clearly to their physicians.

But I also show the pitfalls of this information-heavy approach to medical decision making, pitfalls I've become all too aware of because I have spent time on both ends of the stethoscope. I have not only practiced as a physician, working with patients to make difficult decisions, but I have also been involved in serious medical decisions as a patient and, just as importantly, as a spouse. I have witnessed the limits of information when it comes to fully engaging patients and their families in difficult medical decisions. That's why, in part IV, I show why we won't achieve true, shared decision making unless we make efforts to prepare physicians to interact with prepared patients.

KNOWING WHAT THE OTHER PERSON'S THINKING

I pressed the diaphragm of my stethoscope against Betty Moorman's chest wall. At the gestalt level, I could tell that her heart wasn't beating normally, so I honed in on different phases of her heartbeat. I concentrated on the beginning of the beat, the *lub* in the proverbial *lub-dub*—what we doctors call the S1. Was the S1 regular? Was it distinct from the S2? Was it . . .

PFFHHT BLARGHDIT GLMPH YARG!!!

A sound like a lion with loose dentures ripped through my eardrums. It was the sound of Moorman's voice, amplified by the instrument pressed to her sternum.

The stethoscope is a listening device. Before the stethoscope, doctors listened to patients' lungs and hearts by pressing their ear directly onto their chests. I tried this recently with my wife (yep, we have that kind of relationship), and I have to say the auditory experience wasn't very satisfying.

The stethoscope was designed so that its earplugs would block out external sounds, thereby allowing vibrations inside the patient's chest to be transmitted directly from the diaphragm at the end of the instrument to the listener's ear canals. In other words, it wasn't designed for improving doctor–patient conversations. A patient's voice, transmitted through a stethoscope pressed to his chest, sounds a bit like a Led Zeppelin bass line dialed up to eleven on a broken woofer.

I expect every clinician has had a version of this ear-shattering experience. Hopefully, most respond more graciously than I did that day. Tired from a night of being on-call, I shot a stern look at my patient and shushed her at a volume (given the stethoscope plugged into my ears) that caused her roommate to turn off the television, thinking I was directing my ire her way.

I failed the first test of empathy. I didn't consider that my patient had no idea what her voice sounded like through my medical instrument. I had no excuse. Dozens of patients had made the same mistake with me already. I was painfully aware of the folly of talking while a doctor is listening to one's chest through a stethoscope. But I failed to recognize that, before becoming a doctor, I hadn't known this particular feature of how stethoscopes function. I reacted harshly, thinking my patient was an insensitive fool, when that description better fit me. My patient wasn't a fool and certainly wasn't insensitive. Through no fault of her own, she didn't realize that she should not talk while someone was listening to her heart through a stethoscope. For doctors and patients to make good medical decisions, they need to gain a better understanding of what is going on in the mind of the person at the other end of the stethoscope.

Saying that a prostate cancer diagnosis "isn't bad news" is a failure of empathy, an inability to grasp what a patient feels when receiving such news. Figure-skating analogy? Not my most empathetic moment. If I had truly grasped the way my patient was feeling that day, I wouldn't have pushed him so far beyond his comfort zone.

Assuming your doctor knows when you are scared? That's not going to get you the care you deserve. Nodding along even though your doctor's words sound like a foreign language? Maybe that will save face, but isn't it more important that you understand what she's saying? There is no shame in interrupting your doctor to ask questions.

As I lay out the new world of doctor–patient negotiation—the world of post-paternalistic medicine—I'll show why good decision making depends less on resolving moral dilemmas (like deciding whether to be paternalistic or hands-off) than on getting doctors and patients conversing with each other, making an effort to get a better sense of what the person on the other end of the stethoscope is thinking and feeling. The patient-empowerment movement of the 1970s succeeded in transforming the doctor–patient relationship, but too often it has failed in its ultimate goal of helping patients receive the medical care that best fits their individual preferences. All too frequently it has left both doctors and patients performing a dance they're not limber enough to pull off. Good medical decisions require shared decision making. And many patients and physicians aren't ready to share. I'll show that we can fix this problem. But the fix will require work on both ends of the stethoscope.

PART I

The Rise of the Empowered Patient

ONE
When Doctor Knew Best

With a touch of my hand I silenced my beeper, hoping to finish a quick hallway conversation before returning the page. Thirty seconds later, the beeping resumed—someone clearly wanted to talk to me right away. I answered the page and was soon striding briskly toward the operating room, ready to handle the emergency.

It was 1995 and Catherine Williams lay anesthetized on an operating room table with an open surgical wound, a large throat tumor now visible to the outside world. I am not a surgeon, so they hadn't called me there to assist in her operation. Nor am I an oncologist, an anesthesiologist, or any kind of "ologist" relevant to the care of such a patient. Why then had they rushed me to the O.R.?

Because I was the hospital ethics consultant, and the surgeon faced a moral dilemma.

"Her tumor is more invasive than I thought," he told me. "I assumed from the radiology images that I'd be able to remove it without affecting her speech. But now that I have had a closer look, I can see that the operation will leave her mute."

He had told Williams before the operation that her cancer was incurable but that the operation would prolong her life, delaying the time when the tumor would threaten vital functions like swallowing and speaking. She had opted for the operation in lieu of an immediate referral to hospice care. She wanted to go out with a fight. But the surgeon wasn't sure that her willingness to fight would extend as far as he knew his scalpel would take him: "I don't know if she would have proceeded with the operation if she had known that she would lose the ability to speak."

We could ask her, of course, but the operation was already underway and waking Williams up would mean halting the procedure, packing up the wound, and waiting for the anesthesia to wear off. The operation would be finished for the day, and the surgeon would only be able to continue removing the tumor by bringing her back to the O.R. on another day, exposing her in the meantime to the risk that her open wound would get infected.

"I am almost positive she will want to continue the operation," he explained, "so all that extra risk will be unnecessary."

Two decades earlier, another woman lay asleep on an operating room table, the tissue from her breast lump frozen and under the discerning eye of a surgical pathologist. The diagnosis was clear. The patient had cancer, news that the pathologist quickly relayed to the surgeon, Dr. William Fouty, Chair of Surgery at the National Naval Medical Center in Bethesda, Maryland.

Fouty was aware that, in just a couple of days, the National Cancer Institute (NCI) was going to announce preliminary results of a randomized clinical trial showing that the procedure he had been performing on breast cancer patients for years—the radical mastectomy—was no better at preventing breast cancer recurrence than a much less invasive operation, the modified radical mastectomy. The radical mastectomy had been the cornerstone of breast cancer treatment for decades, but it was brutal. The procedure typically began with removal of the cancerous breast—not just the lump of cancer, but the entire breast. From there, the procedure continued deeper into the woman's chest, with the surgeon cutting through and removing the muscles underlying the breast tissue, including the pectoralis major and its tiny cousin the pectoralis minor. These muscles were removed not because they were visibly invaded by cancer but because they resided so close to the cancer that they could, potentially, be harboring hidden disease. After the breast and muscles were removed, the surgeon would shift attention to nearby lymph nodes, once again removing such tissue even in the absence of obvious metastases. Some surgeons even went so far as to remove nearby bone. Better safe than sorry.

The soon-to-be announced NCI trial would show that all these aggressive dissections were unnecessary, that the radical mastectomy was no better at preventing cancer recurrence than the newer, less aggressive modified radical mastectomy. Now, I want to be clear. The modified radical mastectomy was still an aggressive operation, involving removal of the entire breast as well as nearby lymph nodes. Indeed, later trials would show that many women would do just as well with an even more limited procedure, a lumpectomy. But in 1975 the soon-to-be released NCI trial would shake up the world of surgical oncology, a world dominated by the view that the more tissue sacrificed to the scalpel, the better chance a patient would be cured.

Fouty, however, wasn't shaken up by the impending NCI announcement. He refused to believe that the findings were legitimate. Dismissing the preliminary findings, he proceeded with the more aggressive procedure. As with most surgeons, the logic of the radical mastectomy struck him as obvious. Taking out more local tissue *must* reduce the chance of recurrence. Tumor removal was the key.

Besides, Fouty had received presidential permission to conduct the more aggressive operation. The patient, you see, was Betty Ford, the fifty-two-year-old wife of the president of the United States. Fouty had met with her and the president before conducting the biopsy and had told them that he believed strongly in removing as much local tissue as possible. He also told them that speed was critical—no time to ponder complicated medical facts. The first lady's tumor needed to be diagnosed and treated right away; so quickly, in fact, that Fouty urged a one-step procedure—biopsy and mastectomy on the same day, with no need to wake the first lady up to discuss the biopsy results before proceeding with surgery.

The Fords accepted Fouty's advice. Gerald Ford might have been the most powerful man in the world, but who was he to question the authority of an eminent surgeon like Fouty? Doctor knows best!

That means that when Betty Ford went to sleep to undergo the biopsy, her fate was already out of her hands. The doctors would consult with the president, tell him what they saw in the frozen tissue, and proceed with the operation if they deemed it necessary.

Two operations separated by two decades, but in reality separated by a revolution. In 1995, a surgeon urgently paged an ethicist rather than continue with a procedure that his patient might not want. In 1975, there were no ethics consultants to speak of, nor much recognition that decisions about how to treat diseases like throat cancer or breast cancer involved value judgments, no acknowledgment that the "right" choice often depends on patient preferences. Fouty certainly didn't acknowledge Betty Ford's right to self-determination that day, as he tunneled deep into her armpit, removing any lymph nodes he could find. He didn't wrestle with finding the best way to elicit her preferences or with determining the best way to communicate the facts to her so that she could decide whether to opt for the newer, less invasive procedure. Nor did he, for a moment, behave like someone intimidated by her power or prestige. He behaved like a man in charge. That's probably why, when he first palpated the lump on her breast, he didn't even tell her he had found anything abnormal. He just shrugged and left the examining room. The first lady would only learn that something was wrong when her appointment secretary told her that her primary care physician was coming by with another doctor to see her that night.

Nor did Betty Ford struggle with her role in the decision. In her autobiography, she simply wrote that Fouty "explained to me what this operation would entail," an operation that was presented to her as a fait accompli rather than as an option to consider. Ford was so comfortable in the role of passive patient, in fact, that she wrote almost matter-of-factly about how her primary care doctor, William Lukash, had informed her daughter Susan about the cancerous lump before relaying that information to Ford herself. "Your mother has a lump in her breast," he had told Susan. "There's a good chance it's cancer, and she doesn't know, so hush, hush. Don't say anything to anybody."

Hush, hush indeed.

To understand where we are, we need to know where we came from. To understand, then, how the first lady could have become such a secondary player in her own medical history, we need a quick trip through the history of medical decision making and doctor–patient communication, starting with a rapid tour of ancient Greece.

I SWEAR BY APOLLO

"I swear by Apollo the Physician and Asclepius and Hygieia and Panacea and all the gods and goddesses, that I will fulfill according to my ability and judgment this oath and this covenant."

So begins the most famous document in the history of medical ethics, the Hippocratic oath—a pledge that has been taken in various forms by hundreds of thousands of physicians over the centuries. When the oath was written, it codified the unique moral duties that physicians were expected to accept as inherent to their profession.

And what were those duties?

> To hold him [sorry about that, ladies—it was a man's world back then] who has taught me this art as equal to my parents and to live my life in partnership with him . . .

Medical practice in ancient Greece centered on an apprenticeship model. Thus the oath continues:

And if he is in need of money, to give him a share of mine, and to regard his offspring as equal to my brothers in male lineage and to teach them this art—if they design to learn it—without fee and covenant.

The apprentice was expected to show gratitude to the person who brought him into this field, a field that was, essentially, an exclusive club with special privileges:

To give a share of my precepts and oral instruction and all the other learning to my sons and to the sons of him who has instructed me. And to pupils who have signed the covenant and have taken the oath according to medical law, and to no one else.

You heard that right: "to no one else"! When Betty Ford developed breast cancer, she found herself face-to-face with a two-thousand-year-old tradition of silence. The physicians she encountered inherited a legacy of concealment. In Hippocrates's time, being a physician meant being a member of a secret society. Medical information was for doctors only, not for members of other professions and *certainly* not for patients. Hippocrates never directed doctors to educate their patients or to empower them to make decisions. Instead, he exhorted physicians "to secure the cooperation of their patients." Patients weren't to be informed; they were to be persuaded.

We don't know much about Hippocrates's life. Historians have established that he lived approximately four centuries before the time of Christ, on the Greek island of Kos. Hippocrates's views got him into trouble with authorities. For instance, he believed illness could be explained by the tools of reason and science, a radical belief that so bothered religious leaders—who held that disease was punishment from unhappy gods—they threw him into prison for nearly twenty years. It was during his time in prison that he is believed to have written the medical texts that would establish his fame.

Most of what we know about Hippocrates the man is legend, not fact. We do know that he lived to a ripe old age, but published accounts of him living over 100 years are probably wrong. We don't know much about his family life or his personality. Historians are not even in agreement about which of his attributed writings were actually written by the man himself. But we do have a pretty good idea of how Hippocrates and his contemporaries practiced medicine. We know that physicians were not able to treat most illnesses because of the impoverished state of medical science at the time. Back then, if you were unlucky enough to get sick and hoped to get better, it would be through the efforts of Mother Nature, not those of your physician. Even making an accurate diagnosis would be a stretch for your physician, because the prohibition against human dissection had left physicians largely ignorant of even the most basic anatomy. So the Hippocratean physician focused his efforts on prognostication—on figuring out whether you were going to live or die.

Not that you'd be privy to such prognostications. The goal of all this was not for the physician to communicate such information to the patient in question. Remember that the Hippocratean physician was trained to comfort the patient, and bad news was hardly deemed comforting. Instead of giving patients bad news, then, Hippocrates urged physicians to communicate:

> . . . calmly and adroitly, concealing most things from the patient while you're attending to him. Give necessary orders with cheerfulness and serenity, drawing his attention away from what is being done to him; sometimes reprove sharply and emphatically, and sometimes comfort with solicitude and attention, revealing nothing of the patient's future or present condition.

More than two and a half millennia before Betty Ford was diagnosed with breast cancer, physicians believed that their most important duty was not to involve patients in decisions or even to inform them about the details of their medical conditions but to care for their emotional and physical needs. Determining how to meet those needs—therein lay true medical expertise. With no antibiotics or IV tubes, physicians weren't treating disease as much as observing it, learning from experience where things were likely to go and what they could do to minimize patient suffering.

Modern bioethicists have a word for the moral norm that dominated ancient medical practice: beneficence—actions that are done for the benefit of others. Physicians in ancient times believed that their professional training provided them with unique insight into what was in their patients' best interests. If a patient's symptoms were best relieved by ingesting a specific medicine, the physician's job was only to secure that patient's cooperation. If a dying patient's bliss depended upon remaining ignorant of his prognosis, the physician's duty was to keep the patient in the dark. In all circumstances, it was the doctor's judgment that mattered. As physicians said when reciting the Hippocratic oath, "I will prescribe regimens for the good of my patients according to my ability and judgment." The physician's judgment, not the patient's!

Dr. William Fouty was adhering to the same ancient ethic when he told Betty Ford that if her lump was cancerous, she needed to undergo a radical mastectomy. When he ignored the upcoming NCI announcement and removed Ford's chest muscles, he was beneficently doing what he thought was in her best interest. He gave Betty Ford the same advice he would have given his wife or his mother.

Was he arrogant? Of course he was. We're talking about a famous physician, one who would be called to the bedside of the first lady. Was he exerting his power over the president and first lady? Absolutely. But power in the service of what, in his confident opinion, was best for the patient. Fouty wasn't trying to enrich himself by performing an unnecessarily invasive operation. He wasn't trying to prove that he was more powerful than the president or the first lady. He was just trying to save Ford's life.

THE DAWN OF MEDICAL SCIENCE

In 1928, Alexander Fleming was studying staphylococcal bacteria in his lab, those ubiquitous organisms notorious for causing nasty infections like boils and carbuncles. Fleming's lab was littered with petri dishes, colonies of staphylococci reproducing sinisterly in the clear agar. Nothing in the laboratory or nature was known to halt these rude invaders. But then Fleming went away on holiday one week, leaving the petri dishes unattended, and mold began growing within some of the cultures in his absence, wiping out the staph that had been residing there.

Chance, as they say, favors the prepared mind, and Fleming's mind was quite prepared to appreciate the significance of this discovery. He realized that something in the mold was killing the bacteria. So he isolated the mold and confirmed that it killed staph and other related bacteria. In a happy accident, he had discovered penicillin. But his laboratory finding wouldn't yet revolutionize medical care, because Fleming was not prepared to make clinical use of his discovery—the penicillin molecule was too difficult to produce for him to pursue it any further.

That job was left to a group of biochemists in Australia who isolated the active compound in the mold and purified enough of it to see if it could eradicate real-life infections.

The researchers gathered eight unfortunate laboratory mice and inoculated them with fatal doses of streptococci (a close cousin of staphylococcus). They gave penicillin to four of these mice—the only ones, as it turns out, who survived the night. The young researchers had moved from concept to proof of concept. Penicillin worked! Now they needed to test the drug on an infected human. So they kept their eyes peeled for any patient arriving at their hospital with the kind of infection that could respond to this drug.

They didn't have to wait long. Word reached the doctors that a policeman was losing a battle against a staph infection he had acquired when scratched by a rosebush. They rushed to his bedside and injected him with penicillin. They were ecstatic to observe that his health rapidly improved—his fever abated and his breathing became less labored. But his infection was quite advanced and they quickly exhausted their limited supply of the drug. His symptoms gradually returned. Desperate to keep treating him, they collected his urine, isolated the penicillin that had passed through his system, and reinjected it into his veins. They were once again thrilled to see that he improved. The battle was on. Penicillin injection followed by temporary recovery; relapse followed by urinary recovery of the unmetabolized drug; reinjection and recovery followed by relapse. But with each filtration of his urine, they found themselves with a dwindling supply of the drug. Four days into treatment, they exhausted their supply of penicillin and the policeman succumbed to his infection. Felled by a rosebush.

His death was tragic, but the doctors consoled themselves with the power of their new drug. They had almost succeeded in bringing this man back from the brink. With a larger supply of penicillin, they knew they could have saved his life.

Realizing that British pharmaceutical companies were too busy fulfilling war-related demands, they convinced a U.S. company to produce the drug. The military quickly harnessed the power of penicillin to assist in the Allied war effort. In 1941, soldiers by the thousands were dying of wound-related bacterial infections. Now, one year later, pus-filled battle wounds began melting away in the face of the remarkable antibiotic. Pneumonias that used to kill one out of three infected soldiers were now killing one out of fifteen.

The era of scientifically derived medical treatments had now arrived in full force. But what would this new era mean for how doctors communicated with patients about their medical care? In the prescientific era of medical care, the time of the ancient physicians, there was no point in involving patients in their medical decisions. After all, there were almost no decisions to make. What treatments existed were largely unproven. There weren't scientific trials providing data on, say, the relative risks and benefits of alternative pneumonia therapies.

By the time Fouty took care of Betty Ford in 1975, however, medical science had experienced several decades of remarkable scientific progress. Doctors not only knew how to diagnose most illnesses but could treat many of them too, and in fact had multiple treatment options available for many ills. The miracle of penicillin in the early 1940s was followed by dozens of other miracles. Discoveries raced from laboratory to mouse to bedside at breakneck speed. There was now every reason to involve patients in their medical decisions. But several millennia of tradition had had a way of cementing the habits of both doctors and patients. If the story of medical decision making were linear, then with each medical advance doctors would have had more to talk about with their patients, and the profession would have incrementally shifted from its ethic of beneficence to a more modern ethic of shared decision making. Instead, the dawn of medical science in many respects aggravated the worst features of Hippocratean practice. Rather than build on the ethic of compassion handed to them by their ancient predecessors, modern physicians embraced an ethic of experimentation. Their infatuation with science caused them to expand the code of silence into truly horrific territory.

In the time following World War II, medical practice rapidly shifted from being a diagnostic science to being a therapeutic one. In Hippocrates's time, as we have seen, there was almost no science to medical practice. Doctors were more like religious figures than scientific ones. A doctor's job was not to cure the patient but to console him in his last hours of life, when he was "alone with his patient and God." In this prescientific context, nondisclosure had become a staple of medical practice because physicians so often had so little they could do to alter their patient's trajectory. Telling them the truth in such dire circumstances was simply cruel.

Prior to World War II, medical practice had increasingly become a scientific enterprise. Doctors wielded progressively more sensitive stethoscopes to better diagnose their patients' heart and lung problems. They employed X-rays to better visualize their patients' broken bones and pneumonias. They developed a whole host of powerful interventions that altered the course of illness. Medical researchers eagerly grabbed hold of advances in biology and chemistry and applied them to medical settings. The U.S. government turbocharged these advances by tossing cash at medical researchers through a new agency that would become the National Institutes of Health (NIH). Medical schools quickly became bastions of basic science research, with deans and department chairs increasingly chosen from the ranks of those who had mastered laboratory science at the NIH.

With this growth in the science of medical care came a proliferation of treatment options. Not just one antibiotic but soon two, four, even a dozen. New pills to strengthen hearts, others to lower blood pressure, insulin to control blood sugar, and prednisone to quell inflammation.

Medical schools recruited a new breed of doctors, science wizards who grasped complex mathematical and chemical concepts far better than their college classmates. But this rigorous selection process had an unintended consequence—it contributed to a feeling among those who had made it into the profession that they lived in a world apart from their patients, a rarified world of science and healing their patients could neither enter nor comprehend. If the Hippocratean physician was already a breed apart, a priestlike healer with magical powers, then the new physician-scientist was a breed even further apart. Science, instead of democratizing medical practice, augmented physicians' authority.

With this new authority, and propelled by the rush of medical discoveries, physicians began to see patients as opportunities for scientific advancements, as living laboratories. They began testing out their scientific theories on patients without bothering to inform the patients about their experiments. Saul Krugman laid out this patient-as-laboratory reasoning in a 1959 *New England Journal of Medicine* article. Bemoaning the lack of scientific progress in combating infectious hepatitis, he wrote about the importance of determining the typical progression of symptoms brought on by the virus, the "natural history" of the disease, as doctors call it. "Unfortunately," he wrote, "man is still the only established susceptible host," meaning of course that, if he were going to understand the natural history of the disease, he needed to find humans he could observe from the moment of infection.

But how would Krugman know the exact time any given patient was infected with the hepatitis virus? This is where the story turns sinister. Krugman worked at the Willowbrook State School, an "institution for mentally defective children," as he described it in the journal article. Knowing from experience that these children would inevitably become infected, he purposely inoculated them with the virus and then proceeded to observe them, measuring their blood and analyzing their stools. He made no attempt to get consent from the children's parents.

Following World War II, as physicians embraced the challenge of developing scientific therapies, many of them became willing to cause suffering among their patients in order to advance scientific knowledge. Chester Southam, for instance, could think of no better way to understand the natural history of cancer than by injecting live cancer cells into demented nursing home patients and following the course of their illness. Captain Alton J. Morris, a member of the U.S. Air Force, deemed it completely acceptable to determine the natural history of strep throat by allowing half of his air force colleagues to go untreated while the rest received sulfa drugs, new antibiotics that were known to cure strep. Many of those untreated airmen would develop rheumatic fever, an inflammatory reaction to the strep organism that can cause neurologic damage and heart failure.

Throughout the '50s and '60s nary a month would pass without a major medical journal publishing a study involving surreptitious experiments on human guinea pigs. These experiments were reported in leading medical journals not as case studies of unethical practice, nor as exposés of researchers gone wild. They were unquestioningly published as ho-hum research articles; descriptions of the research methods sat right smack in the middle of each article, unabashedly laying out the deceptions and nondisclosures central to the science at hand, with no one—no editors, no reviewers—raising an eyebrow.

These studies strike our modern sensibilities as being grossly immoral. Yet physicians of the day didn't share this view; they saw themselves as members of an elite group, privy to specialized scientific knowledge, even *discovering* new knowledge in the course of their work. Drawn to medicine in part by its intellectual challenges, this new breed of physicians lived in a different intellectual universe than their largely unscientific patient population, a population that couldn't be expected to understand the scientific method.

Physicians were on what they deemed to be a noble quest, to understand health and sickness in the hope that all of humanity would benefit. Undoubtedly, many of these physicians were driven by ego and fame, but they were also driven by the old Hippocratic ethic of beneficence—making decisions based on their own judgment of what was in their patients' best interests. But "patients" in this case meant future patients, not the ones in their experiments. The Hippocratic ethic, of caring compassionately for the individual patient, had been savagely twisted into a new form. The doctor-as-scientist cared not for the patient on the other end of his stethoscope but for the *world* of future patients who'd benefit from the knowledge gained at the current patient's expense.

To paint broad strokes about medical practice in the '50s and '60s, start with the ancient tradition. The modern physician inherited an ethic of silence, of nondisclosure. This ethic is troubling to twenty-first-century minds, but at least it was an ethic grounded in concern for the interests of individual patients. The Hippocratean physician was perhaps, in retrospect, too secretive with his patients, but at least he was focused on relieving a patient's suffering. By the mid-twentieth century many physicians, caught up in a wave of discoveries, had embraced the worst part of the Hippocratean tradition—the silence—and abandoned the best—the focus on promoting the best interests of the individual patient. These medical researchers had lost sight of traditional ethical boundaries.

They got away with these unethical practices because the general public viewed physicians with incredible deference. Laypeople were reluctant to question the decisions these doctors made on behalf of science. Most patients were happy to remain ignorant about their medical care, content in the belief that their physicians would do what was best. Even as late as 1969, when television producers looked to create a popular medical drama, they turned to Robert Young, famous for having played the lead character in the beloved sitcom *Father Knows Best.* His casting wasn't a coincidence. Marcus Welby, M.D., the title character he played on what would be the number one show in the 1970–71 season, was a man you could trust, the kind of gentle person who fit the day's stereotype of a physician. Contrast Welby with the snarling cynicism of Dr. Gregory House from the hit Fox show of today. According to David Shore, one of the creators of the *House, M.D.* series, he wanted to build the show around a realistic physician, the kind he had encountered while sick in the hospital: "I knew, as soon as they left the room, they would be mocking me relentlessly [for my cluelessness], and I thought it would be interesting to see a character who did that before [he] left the room."

Physician experimenters also felt empowered to treat their patients like guinea pigs because their patients passively accepted whatever medical recommendations their doctors gave them. This deference to physicians was not limited to people's attitudes toward medical researchers. It also shaped the way patients interacted with non-research physicians who, in their crisp white coats, still looked like scientists to most of their patients. If you doubt this statement, consider the unfortunate story of Irma Natanson, whose blind trust in her doctor left her permanently and grotesquely disfigured, mere inches away from an unnecessary death.

THERAPEUTIC PRACTICES

Twenty years before Betty Ford developed breast cancer, Irma Natanson underwent a radical mastectomy to remove a tumor discovered in her left breast. After recovering from the operation, she met with Dr. John Kline, a physician from Wichita, Kansas, who practiced in the emerging specialty of radiation therapy. He told her that the mastectomy had removed every bit of visible tumor but that, on the off chance that microscopic tumor cells were lurking in the area, she would nevertheless benefit from a course of cobalt therapy. He explained to Natanson that she would need to come to the hospital for several weeks of treatment. He patiently showed Natanson where on her body he would point the radiation beams: at her breastbone to treat any residual mammary cells and at nearby lymph nodes in her armpit to disable any cancer cells that had migrated in that direction. He explained that he would devote sixteen sessions to irradiating the area above her left clavicle and twenty-three sessions to targeting her chest wall. He even introduced her to the physicist who would calculate the proper dose of radiation for each region of her body.

Natanson began receiving treatment that very same day. Her case, after all, was fairly routine. Kline explained that while the cobalt treatment was "not without risks," it had been well tolerated by most of his patients.

In the mid-1950s, when Kline treated Natanson, cobalt therapy was relatively new, with so little cobalt available for clinical use that Kline was forced to obtain supplies from the Atomic Energy Commission. Cobalt emits pure gamma rays, an intense dose of radiation by any account and one that could make a person wonder what Kline had meant when he'd said the treatment was "not without risks." But Natanson had no such concerns that day. She deferred to Kline, who clearly understood things about radiation that she'd never grasp. She would come to regret this deference.

Kline's goal was to irradiate Natanson to the verge of tissue viability. That was how radiation treatment worked—it destroyed tissue. The trick was to destroy cancer cells without wiping out healthy bone, muscle, skin, and cartilage. Kline knew he was taking a calculated risk with Natanson's treatment. Unfortunately, he didn't share most of that information with Natanson. He didn't tell her that in a small proportion of cases the treatment permanently damages healthy tissue. Nor did he tell her that the treatment was largely unproven. No surprise there. At the time, almost no medical treatment had been subjected to randomized clinical trials. Doctors like Kline were confident in the merits of the treatments not because said treatments had been scientifically proven but because the treatments made so much damn sense. How could cancer recurrence not be reduced by blasting the tumor site with radiation?

We're near the gloomy end of this story. Natanson dutifully underwent the radiation treatment. All went well, at first, but her radiation burns did not settle down as expected. Her skin became red and inflamed, **and then** it began to break down. So too did the bone and cartilage lying beneath her breast. Her ribs became necrotic—they died and were reabsorbed by her body. In effect, her chest sloughed off her body. It would take the work of a very talented plastic surgeon to pull enough healthy skin up over her chest wall to close the radiation wound. Even then, with her ribs absent, her skin would visibly shudder with each beat of her heart.

Natanson experienced a horrific outcome from her radiation therapy, but what makes her story even more tragic is that her outcome was predictably horrific. Most women didn't suffer as much tissue breakdown as Natanson, but her outcome wasn't unprecedented. When Kline began irradiating Natanson's chest, he knew there was a small chance things could turn out this way; that's why he told her the treatment was "not without risks." He simply decided, unilaterally, that giving her more detail about those risks was unnecessary. And good patient that she was, in keeping with the norms of the day, Natanson didn't ask him to explain these risks. What, after all, would be the point of that? Kline had already decided how to treat her cancer. Further questioning would simply seem pushy.

Kline was not a researcher enrolling unwitting patients in harmful experiments. He was a busy clinician providing routine therapy for a standard diagnosis. And Natanson wasn't a guinea pig being unwittingly enrolled in a scientific experiment. She was just a routine patient, obediently receiving standard therapy. Natanson's treatment complications were unusual but her treatment wasn't. She received doses Kline had prescribed to dozens of patients. She had simply been one of the unlucky ones.

Kline was behaving like most doctors of the day, helping his patient by providing a treatment he believed in ardently without worrying her over unlikely risks. Consider a 1953 survey of doctors in Philadelphia that inquired about what information physicians typically communicated to patients with terminal cancer. A vast majority said they kept their patients in the dark, withholding information about their diagnoses in order to promote their mental health. Such practices were not unique to Philadelphia, the city W. C. Fields quipped he'd spent a year in "one Sunday." In 1960, 84 percent of Chicago-area physicians said they commonly withheld cancer diagnoses from their patients when the prognosis was "grave."

How could they remain silent in the face of such obvious disease? By disclosing misleading information—telling one patient that he has a "growth," telling another he has a "suspicious lesion." More often the cause of the patient's illness was simply not discussed, and the patient was told that everything would work out if they just followed doctors' orders. Telling is "the cruelest thing in the world," said one physician who participated in the Chicago survey. Beneficence demanded silence. Compassion trumped disclosure.

TWO SLEEPING WOMEN

I began this chapter describing two women put under anesthesia so that a surgeon could remove their respective cancers. In 1975, Betty Ford was operated upon by a surgeon confident that he knew what was best for her, and neither she nor her powerful husband were inclined to disagree. Such was the esteem with which physicians were held at the time that almost no one was prepared to question their authority, not even the man who had inherited the presidency of the United States from Richard Nixon.

A mere two decades later, a surgeon was so unsure whether he should continue with an operation that he urgently paged me, then working as an on-call ethicist, to help decide whether to wake up a woman before removing the rest of her cancer and thereby extinguishing her ability to speak. With little coaxing, the surgeon broke off the operation and sent her to the recovery room. When she awoke, she was surprised to learn that he hadn't removed her tumor but grateful that he'd given her a chance to change course. As he had predicted, she chose to continue the operation. But now she was able to enter the procedure with the knowledge of what that procedure would entail and with some final words for her husband, who would never hear her voice again.

Over the course of two and a half millennia, silence dominated medical practice. And now, two decades after Betty Ford's operation, surgeons were requesting ethics consults? What happened so quickly to transform medical decision making?

In part, the revolution in medical practice was simply a sign of the times. By the mid-1970s, authority figures throughout Western society were being challenged by an increasingly restless populace. Civil rights activists were proving that powerless people can become powerful; pacifists were showing that military guns couldn't stand up to public opinion; and feminists were beginning to challenge the naturalness of leaving the world's oversight in the hands of men. Indeed, almost at the same time Betty Ford was undergoing her surgery, feminists were transforming breast cancer care. Concerned that male doctors were needlessly deforming women, they voiced their concerns in magazines and on newscasts about the unnecessary horrors of the radical mastectomy. Some even played an important role in convincing researchers to collect better data about the pros and cons of this unproven surgery.

But it wouldn't be feminists, civil rights activists, or any other "ists" who would give the medical revolution its biggest push. That job was undertaken by a pair of ardent Roman Catholics who would have never considered questioning authority, if it hadn't been for the love of their daughter.

TWO

A Sleeping Girl Wakes Up a Profession

"Mrs. Quinlan, I am authorized to offer you $100,000 for a photograph of your daughter."

The tiny woman hesitated, unsure how to respond politely to this audacious request. She pulled herself together and replied calmly, "I'm sorry, but Karen would never want anyone to see her like this."

Undaunted, the photographer persisted. "Actually, $100,000 is only a starting figure. We could go higher."

In 1975, $100,000 was an almost unprecedented amount of money for a photograph. But no doubt the picture, if the photographer had been able to obtain it, would have fetched far more than that from interested news agencies. Its proposed subject, Karen Ann Quinlan, was perhaps the most famous living twenty-one-year-old on the planet, if, that is, you believed she was alive.

The Quinlans' saga had begun months earlier with a 2 A.M. phone call:

"Is this Mrs. Quinlan?" a woman had asked.

"Yes."

"I'm sorry to tell you, but your daughter is in the hospital. She's in a serious condition, unconscious."

At the time of the phone call, Karen was twenty-one years old and had recently left home to share a place with two young men, a situation that didn't please her conservative Roman Catholic parents. But given the times—the year 1975—they knew their daughter could have been doing far worse things.

Earlier that evening, Karen had had a couple of gin and tonics with friends and had taken a small dose of, among other things, Valium, but not enough alcohol or pharmaceuticals to explain her subsequent condition. Her friends were surprised to see her staggering around as if she were on a real bender. It was very uncharacteristic of Karen. Perhaps the problem was that she had gone on a starvation diet recently, in an effort to get into bikini shape for an upcoming trip to Florida. Maybe with so little food in her system she was more sensitive to the drinks and pills.

Whatever the cause of her drunken-like state, her friends had tucked her into bed confident she'd sleep it off with, at most, a minor hangover. Their confidence couldn't have been more misplaced. Just a couple of hours later they returned to Karen's room and discovered that she wasn't breathing. They called for an ambulance and performed inexpert CPR. Karen would never regain consciousness. Her body had gone without oxygen too long, causing devastatingly irreversible brain damage.

It would be a while before the irreversibility of Karen's condition became apparent. And it would be even longer before the full impact of her plight had ricocheted through the world of medical decision making. Quinlan's case would become the most famous and arguably the most important battle in what was becoming a broad effort to empower patients and families faced with difficult medical decisions. Her family would fight for control of Karen's medical care, a battle that would jump-start the right-to-die movement, spur the growth of the bioethics profession, and force the medical community to realize "medical" decisions would never be purely medical again.

But as Karen's mother, Julia, hung up the phone that night, revolution was the last thing on anyone's mind.

PERSISTENT. VEGETATIVE.

By the time Julia and Joe Quinlan made it to the hospital in nearby Newton, New Jersey, Karen was lying in intensive care, a ventilator tube expertly inserted through her windpipe, IV tubes snaking out from underneath the bedcovers. Eyes closed, she lay there motionless, no sign of injury apparent on her slender frame, but no obvious signs of alertness either. Julia and Joe stayed by her bedside, praying, confident that God would help their daughter recover.

A few days into the hospital stay, it appeared their prayers had been answered. Karen began to move her head, rotating it slowly from side to side. Then she opened her eyes. The first stirrings of consciousness? "Karen!" her father shouted excitedly. But Karen didn't seem to recognize either of her parents. Her eyes stared vacantly into space, as if she were blind.

Several days passed with no signs that Karen was waking up. Now in over their heads, the doctors at Newton brought in Dr. Robert Morse, a neurologist from nearby St. Clare's Hospital, arguably the most prestigious hospital in that part of New Jersey. Morse strode into the ICU with confidence that belied his mere six years of clinical experience. He examined Karen, looked over her records, and came to a conclusion. He told the distraught parents that he was optimistic about Karen's chance of recovery, but only if they transferred her to St. Clare's, where they could make use of the latest in medical technology.

The ensuing weeks proved Morse's optimism to be unfounded. Karen didn't recover. Instead, the damage to her motor cortex began wreaking havoc upon her neuromuscular system. Her body was now rigid, her feet and hands curled up tightly, like a child grabbing on to a piece of candy. The muscles in the front of her neck had clamped down in what looked like a painful spasm, pitching her head forward unnaturally. She had recently begun exhibiting sleep–wake cycles, but the waking parts of her days weren't accompanied by any kind of awareness. Instead, when she was "awake," her head would move side to side at random intervals, her mouth either contorted into a painful-looking grimace or locked open in what resembled an endless scream. It looked to Karen's parents like she was in pain, but the doctors assured them that she couldn't feel a thing.

On May 25, a month and a half after Karen had lost consciousness, Dr. Morse explained to Karen's parents that her situation had become dire. She was no longer showing signs of coming out of the coma. Karen, he told them, would never again have a sentient thought. She had entered into what physicians called PVS, a persistent vegetative state.

The term PVS was coined in 1972, only three years before Karen's accident, by a pair of physicians who had been studying various states and stages of coma. *Vegetative* is a word medical experts use when referring to unconscious bodily functions, such as digestion and circulation, which take place involuntarily. Such functions contrast with more voluntary processes, like throwing a softball or solving a crossword puzzle. Applied to someone like Karen, the term PVS meant to imply that all of her functions—not just digestion but even her facial grimaces—were involuntary. As Morse explained to Karen's parents, her cerebral cortices had been so damaged that she no longer had the capacity to be conscious. More primitive brain functions were still working, to control her heart rate and blood pressure, for instance, and to initiate the sleep–wake cycles they had been witnessing. Many basic reflexes were intact too, which explained why her eyes darted briefly in the direction of loud noises. But Karen wasn't hearing those noises; she wasn't responding to the sounds. The light of consciousness was permanently extinguished. They'd never speak with their beautiful daughter again.

Morse, the expert, was kindly and gently helping the grieving family understand Karen's situation. Hippocrates would have been proud. Morse was using his medical knowledge to help people come to terms with a loved one's prognosis. Now they just had to accept his conclusion.

COMING TO TERMS

Julia Quinlan must have worked her way through her rosary beads hundreds of times over those long, painful days, pleading with God to bring her daughter back to life. But even in the midst of her prayers, she was open to the idea that God had a plan. Maybe Karen wasn't destined to survive this ordeal. Julia thought back to all the times Karen had spoken to family and friends about dying young, even telling her parents to donate her eyes to an eye bank if something happened to her. Morse's grim prognostications were a bitter pill to swallow, but swallow them she did nonetheless. She knew he was right. Karen would never be Karen again.

But her husband Joe was slower to give up hope. He would sit at Karen's bedside talking to her, always looking for signs that she was understanding his words. At one point late that spring, he became obsessed by the idea of moving Karen to Arizona, thinking that the desert air would revive her. He pleaded with the doctors to get her off the ventilator so that he could transfer Karen to a hospital in Arizona. Both Morse and the ICU physician recognized that Joe's Arizona dreams were fantastical. However, they also agreed that the time had arrived to wean Karen from the ventilator.

So strange to hear that word, *wean*. We usually associate that word with the life-giving milk mothers provide to their babies. Mothers don't wean babies from their milk in order for those babies to die. They wean them to move them on in their lives, toward bigger and better things. Julia Quinlan had never had the chance to wean Karen as a baby, because they had adopted her. Now the doctors wanted to get rid of the breathing machine, that cold mechanical object sitting by her bedside, and they called it weaning?

The ICU team explained how they would proceed in weaning Karen from the ventilator. The ventilator tubes ran from the machine to a hole—a tracheotomy site—that surgeons had made in the front of Karen's neck. With this tracheotomy in place, the doctors explained, they would not need to pull the breathing tube out of Karen's windpipe, as they would normally do with patients after surgery. Instead, they could simply detach the tube from a connector positioned on her trachea. That way if Karen stopped breathing, they could quickly reattach the ventilator as simply as clipping a leash on a dog's collar (although they didn't use that analogy).

The moment arrived. They separated Karen from her breathing tube. The weaning had begun. If she tired too much from breathing on her own, the doctors were prepared to reattach Karen's ventilator for a while and give her, literally, a breather. Which is what they did several times over the ensuing hours. But soon they recognized a pattern in Karen's breathing. When in her awake cycles, Karen could breathe on her own. That was a good sign. But once she entered a sleep cycle, she would stop breathing. Joe's hopes of weaning his daughter from the ventilator were dashed.

That's when it hit him. His daughter was dying; maybe she was dead already. The only thing keeping her from going to heaven, he realized, was the ventilator. He could not remain in denial any longer. He realized the only humane thing to do was to withdraw Karen from the ventilator so that she could die with grace and dignity. He talked things over with Julia and learned that she had arrived at the same conclusion a while ago. They were now in complete agreement. The two parents asked to meet with the medical team, finally ready to hand their daughter over to God's care.

THE END OF THE BEGINNING

The Quinlans met with Dr. Morse on July 31, with the hospital chaplain Father Pat in attendance. Joe was so emotional he spoke at half volume. "Since the doctors can't help Karen," he said, "and they're convinced she's going to die, it is our decision and wish that she be removed from the ventilator and returned to a natural state."

Julia spoke in support of her husband's passionate statement, stating with grim finality, "She would never want to be kept alive this way."

Morse seemed to understand. He put his hand on Joe's shoulder. "I think you've made the right decision." One of the ICU nurses ran to the administrative offices to grab paperwork, releasing the hospital from liability in causing Karen's death. Everything was set.

Until the next morning, when Dr. Morse called Joe and blurted out that he had a "moral problem with the decision." He needed time to think things through. The Quinlans were shocked, but no more so than the following day, when Morse called them again, an air of steely determination now in his voice. "Mr. Quinlan," he said (dropping the more informal "Joe" that he had used in previous conversations), "I find that I will not do it."

The doctor had made *his* decision, and in his mind the controversy was over. As he saw it, doctors are charged with saving patients' lives and granted authority by society to make difficult medical decisions for their patients. Morse had medical training that the Quinlans did not. They had stated their opinion to him about how they wanted him to care for their daughter, but the final decision lay with him, and he wouldn't withdraw a ventilator from a twenty-one-year-old woman who would die as a result of his action. Ain't. Gonna. Happen.

The nation was about to be caught up in a power struggle between a well-intentioned physician and two parents whose love for their daughter trumped their respect for authority.

THE TWILIGHT OF AUTHORITY

The decade preceding the Quinlans' plight had not been a good one for authority figures. The police? The military? No longer were they held up in universal esteem by an adoring public. Even the authority of the president had been turned asunder, with Nixon resigning less than a year before Karen's accident.

But the Quinlans were not antiauthoritarian by any stretch of the imagination. Joe was a decorated war veteran who had lost a hand at the Battle of the Bulge. His time in the military had taught him the importance of hierarchy and order. Julia, for her part, could have been cast as the housewife next door in a *Leave It to Beaver* episode. Not a feminist in any way, shape, or form, she was a mother and a wife foremost, never stepping outside traditional gender expectations. Not that she lacked leadership qualities. She was president of her church rosary society. Both Quinlans, in fact, were deeply involved in the Roman Catholic Church, an organization with a strong authority ethic that felt comfortable to them. Before deciding whether to ask the doctors to remove Karen's ventilator, they each had spoken at length with their priest to find out whether such an action would be consistent with Church teachings. Yes, they were told, the Church does not require doctors to keep patients alive by extraordinary means.

The Quinlans were quite respectful of physician authority too. Up until that point in Karen's care, they had let the doctors make all of the decisions, not even asking questions when they didn't understand what their doctors were doing or saying. Up until then, in fact, it seemed as if the doctors had involved them in a wide array of decisions. The doctors would explain what was happening to Karen's body—maybe a fever, perhaps pneumonia—then the doctors would propose a course of action—some antibiotics, say, or a change of an IV line—and the Quinlans would nod. "Yes, of course, Doctor. Do what you think is best." And the doctors would happily proceed, permission now granted.

But now, when the Quinlans had finally made their agonizing decision—backed up by the authority of their church and the strength of their moral convictions—the doctors had said no. Their permission was no longer relevant. Julia was stunned. "All along, we've been signing permission slips for all the tests you took, all the surgeries, every little thing you ever did for Karen. You've asked us to sign papers before you'd do it. Why is it now, all of a sudden, our permission isn't good enough?" The doctors had been in charge all along, not the parents.

The Quinlans felt backed into a corner. Not inclined to be trouble-makers, and not the kind of people searching high and low for social causes, they nevertheless felt compelled to act. They didn't have a cause; they had a daughter. And if their daughter was going to be al-lowed to die a natural death, they needed a lawyer.

SEEING GHOSTS

Lawyers had had precious little success overturning medical tradi-tion prior to the Quinlan case, even lawyers who had held seats in the U.S. Senate. In 1968, Senator Walter Mondale had called upon a score of the most eminent physicians in the world to testify to the Senate Committee on Government Operations about the ethical and social implications of medical advances, especially in the new field of organ transplantation. Dr. John Najarian, a pioneer in liver transplantation from the University of Minnesota, spoke to this committee, as did Norman Shumway, an innovative heart surgeon from Stanford Uni-versity. But the true rock star of the proceedings was Christiaan Bar-nard, the photogenic South African surgeon who just three months earlier had performed the very first human heart transplant.

Mondale's goal was to establish the groundwork for a national com-mission in charge of overseeing controversial medical decisions, the kind that raised broad societal questions doctors were not capable of addressing on their own. His plan at the hearings was to ask tough questions that would force physicians to acknowledge their inability to make these decisions alone.

But Barnard would have none of it. "You are seeing ghosts where there are no ghosts," he told Mondale. Establish such a commission, he said, and the burden of federal regulation would cause the United

States to be at a competitive disadvantage. "I will go so far ahead, they will never catch up with me."

That remark hit home for the U.S. surgeons gathered there that day. Shumway, for example, had trained Barnard when they were both at the University of Minnesota, and now he was watching his former pupil exceed his own accomplishments.

But Mondale wasn't worried about competition between doctors for fame. He was concerned that organ transplantation was creating dilemmas beyond the expertise of physicians to resolve. Organ allocation, for instance: How should society determine which patients should receive transplantable organs when they became available?

"This decision should be made by doctors," Barnard opined, "as they have made the same decisions in the past." When pushed for a fuller explanation, Barnard did not back down. "I do not think that the public is qualified to make these decisions . . . You must leave it in the people's hands who are capable of doing it."

Barnard was not used to being questioned by anyone about his medical decision making. His patients trusted him completely, accepted his word as gospel. When he spoke with Louis Washkansky, for instance, about receiving what would be the world's first heart transplant, neither patient nor surgeon felt any need to second-guess the wisdom of the surgery. "Mr. Washkansky, I have come to introduce myself," Barnard had said. "We intend on doing a heart transplant on you, and for this you will be admitted to my ward."

"That's fine with me. I'm ready and waiting for it."

"If you like, I can tell you what we know and don't know about this," said Barnard. "We know you have a heart disease for which we can do nothing more. You have had all possible treatment, and you are getting no better. We can put a normal heart into you, after taking out your heart that's no longer any good, and there's a chance you can get back a normal life again."

"So they told me. I'm ready to go ahead."

As Barnard recounts this story, the patient said no more and his eyes remained fixed on Barnard's with no indication (as Barnard interpreted the situation) that he wanted to know any more. So Barnard returned his glance and said, "Well then, good-bye."

Their conversation was over. It was time for the world's first heart transplant.

Such was a physician's authority in 1968. Called in front of U.S. senators, they were adamant about who was in charge of making what they saw as purely medical decisions.

The world was beginning to ask questions, but they weren't having much success in curbing physician authority. Mondale's hearings, other than creating a few headlines, went nowhere. It would take seven years to turn the tide against physicians' unquestioned authority, and it was not senators who did the turning. It was the Quinlans.

THE WORLD WATCHES

Joe Quinlan had left for work thirty minutes earlier, so when the doorbell rang at 8 A.M., Julia was curious about who would be dropping by at such an early hour. Still in her robe, she politely opened the door and a thin young man introduced himself. "Hello, I'm Arnold Diaz from CBS." Word had gotten out that the Quinlans were taking St. Clare's Hospital to court and the media storm had begun. Television, radio, and newspaper reporters flocked to New Jersey from around the globe to track the fate of the sleeping beauty.

The Quinlan's story struck a nerve. Several nerves, in fact. First, there was the victim—a beautiful twenty-one-year-old "girl," who lay in bed in the mysterious space between dead and alive. Prior to the Quinlans' lawsuit, the general public had never heard about her strange diagnosis, of being in a persistent vegetative state. Now they were learning that Karen was sometimes "awake" but never conscious. The public was half confused and two-thirds mesmerized.

Then there was the ventilator. This relatively new technology was confusing to most laypeople, especially in the context of chronic respiratory failure. A ventilator in an operating room was a temporary, invisible intervention. But for a ventilator to be sitting there at Karen's bedside day after day, literally sustaining her life—that was something most people had not realized was a possibility. People's reaction to this breathing machine resonated with discomfort. *Time* magazine characterized the ventilator in almost criminal terms: "Her [Karen's] body convulses slightly every few seconds as an artificial respirator, surgically connected to her windpipe, forces her lungs to work." The words are telling—"artificial" not natural, "forces" not assists.

The Quinlans were also put off by this piece of high-tech equipment. Julia called it "that grey console called the respirator." She would add, "It seems like such a cold machine." The media was entranced: the warm body of a young woman, kept alive against the wishes of her parents by a cold, unfeeling ventilator. That left the media with what seemed to be the biggest part of the story, the unresolved debate about the morality of disconnecting the ventilator. Would such an act be homicide? Was Joe Quinlan, by asking the court to make him Karen's legal guardian so that he could direct the doctors to disconnect the ventilator, in effect trying to play God? Or was it the *doctors* who were playing God, keeping alive a body that ten years earlier would have perished for lack of medical technology?

The newspapers were filled with quotes from strange new creatures called ethicists—philosophers, theologians, and lawyers who were being asked to explain the difference between homicide and euthanasia, between killing someone and letting someone die, and between ordinary and extraordinary means. Most of these ethicists were professors ensconced in the arts and humanities departments of their respective universities. The Quinlan case brought them out of their ivory towers to help the nation wrestle with the very troubling questions raised by her situation. By the end of Karen's story, the bioethics movement had been catapulted into the corridors of the hospital. (In fact, by the time I went to medical school a decade later, my medical school had joined many others in having a philosopher on its faculty and an ethics committee on call 24/7.)

Ventilator, respirator; euthanasia, homicide; artificial, natural—all kinds of controversial new topics, but underlying all the debates was a much more momentous question: Whose job is it to make these decisions?

DOCTORS IN COURT

In the previous chapter, I relayed the unfortunate story of Irma Natanson, whose flesh dissolved after exposure to beams of cobalt radiation. Natanson's story is a famous one in the history of medical decision making because she sued her doctor for negligence, but not the usual kind of negligence. Not for making a mistake, for instance, in dosing her cobalt. Not even for being negligent in deciding that her condition might benefit from this treatment. Instead, she sued her doctor for being negligent in *informing* her about the risks of the treatment—for not involving her, the patient, in the decision. Natanson had had no idea that cobalt treatment carried even a remote chance of causing significant problems. All she had heard from her doctor was that it was the latest and best treatment and that, while the therapy would be long and arduous, things would work out fine in the end. How could she properly consent to a therapy that had never been fully described?

In a landmark decision, the court hearing Natanson's case in 1960 decided that Dr. Kline's lack of communication had crossed over into negligence. In justifying its conclusion, the Kansas Supreme Court asserted that patients have a right to be involved in their medical decisions. "Anglo-American law starts with the premise of thoroughgoing self-determination," the opinion stated and continued (in the gendered language of the day), "Each man is considered to be master of his own body."

A thrilling bit of language, which seemed to assert that patients will now be given equal footing in their medical decisions. But despite framing the issue as one of patient self-determination, the court was not ready to put patients at equal standing with physicians. That, after all, would amount to a court second-guessing physicians about what is best for their patients. The Kansas Supreme Court wrote, "The duty of the physician to disclose is limited to those disclosures which a reasonable medical practitioner would make under the same or similar circumstances." And how are doctors supposed to figure out whom to tell what? According to the justices, that was "primarily a question of medical judgment."

The courts exhibited similar deference to physician judgment twelve years later, when considering the unfortunate case of Jerry Canterbury, a nineteen-year-old FBI clerk troubled by back pain caused by what his doctors suspected was a ruptured disc. The doctors had injected dye into the fluid surrounding Jerry's spinal cord, a procedure called a myelogram, and noticed an area where the dye was unable to flow, a filling defect that confirmed their suspicions of a ruptured disc. Jerry was examined by a neurosurgeon, Dr. William Spence, who concluded that the young man needed surgery. He called Jerry's mother on the phone and she expressed her concerns, asking the surgeon if the operation was serious. He deflected her concerns: "Not any more than any other operation."

The operation went well, but the recovery was a disaster. Left unattended in his hospital room while attempting to empty his bladder, Jerry fell down and injured his tender spinal cord. He suffered permanent neurologic damage, which would interfere with normal bowel and bladder functions and leave him temporarily unable to walk.

His mother sued the neurosurgeon and the hospital for failing to adequately inform her about the risks of the treatment. The judge hearing the case felt badly for the young man, who now "hobbles about on crutches, a victim of the paralysis of bowel and urinary incontinence." The judge was also displeased at the lack of information given to this young man and his family, concluding that true consent "is the informed exercise of a choice, and that entails an opportunity to evaluate knowledgably the options available and the risks attendant upon each."

But Judge Spottswood Robinson was still unwilling to question the neurosurgeon's authority to determine what information patients really needed in order to make these decisions. While on the one hand he seemed to side with patients, writing that "respect for the patient's right of self-determination on particular therapy demands a standard set by law for physicians rather than one which physicians may or may not impose upon themselves," with the other hand he took patients' rights away, writing that "when medical judgment enters the picture . . . prevailing medical practice must be given its just due."

And what would qualify as "just due"? Judge Robinson never spelled that out.

The Natanson and Canterbury lawsuits are still taught in U.S. law schools today as landmarks in establishing patients' rights to self-determination but rights, as we have seen, that still took a backseat to physician judgment. Patient advocates had scaled the castle wall only to be rebuffed. It was this legal climate that the Quinlans encountered when they sued to take decision-making authority away from Karen's uncooperative doctors.

THEIR DAY IN COURT

The Quinlans were represented by Paul Armstrong, an idealistic young lawyer so compelled by their situation that he quit his low-paying job in legal aid and went without income for the several months it took to argue their case. Their first stop in the legal system (and each side was committed to an appeal, if the initial decision was unfavorable) was in front of the bench of New Jersey Superior Court Judge Robert Muir. Armstrong presented a strong case for his clients. "I suggest," he stated to Muir, with an air of confidence that belied his true emotional state, "that the answer to the tragedy of Karen Ann Quinlan is to be found in the love, faith, and courage of her family, who ask only that she be allowed to return to God with grace and dignity."

But Armstrong was opposed by a slew of lawyers. There was the court-appointed guardian, Daniel Coburn, for instance. (Joe Quinlan was suing not to force Karen's doctors to remove her ventilator but to be named legal guardian for his daughter, a position denied him by the hospital and courts so far because of the controversy over Karen's treatment.) Coburn argued that it wasn't up to Karen's father to decide what to do, nor was it up to the court, for that matter. Even God was irrelevant, in Coburn's view. "God's will," he said, "takes second place to what medical science will do for her." Coburn was adamant that disconnecting the ventilator would amount to euthanasia, a belief that was vehemently echoed in the testimony of Morris County prosecutor Donald Collester.

But the hospital team had a more important goal in mind than squabbling over the definition of euthanasia or determining the proper way to care for patients with PVS. Much more crucially, they wanted to re-establish that those decisions—about how to care for such patients, about the very morality of withdrawing ventilators— were best made by physicians. As a matter of fact, when Karen's neurologist, Dr. Morse, was asked to comment on the Roman Catholic view of extraordinary means, he couldn't resist critiquing this theology despite his own strong Catholic views. He questioned whether "the Church had some medical support to make their decision on. That is what we were trying to find out. It was on that basis that I would have considered—if there was some medical tradition that would support the case, other than brain death."

In Morse's view, the Church was extending its moral authority into a medical arena that it neither controlled nor understood. He concluded his testimony with a terse summary of his position: "I cannot break medical tradition."

DEATH BY ANY OTHER NAME

My primary focus in relaying the Quinlan story is to illustrate the battle that took place over who should make medical decisions. But the court was interested in other issues too, none perhaps more profound than the question of whether Karen, with her brain so severely damaged, was still alive. Yet even that topic revealed the reach of physician authority over issues that extended far beyond medical expertise.

In his testimony during the Quinlan trial, the hospital attorney wondered whether medical science would classify Karen as dead, thus ending any concern that extubating her—discontinuing her ventilation—would amount to criminal homicide. Just seven years earlier, a committee of physicians at Harvard had proposed a definition of brain death, designed to help doctors determine whether patients whose hearts and lungs were supported by medical technology were nevertheless deceased. The Harvard criteria had already been legally recognized in eight states, but not in New Jersey. It was these criteria that enabled transplant surgeons to take healthy organs from patients whose heart and lungs were still functioning but whose brains had been virtually destroyed by trauma or injury.

Before the Harvard committee had laid out their criteria, death was a relatively straightforward diagnosis. If a person stopped breathing and lacked a heartbeat, he or she was probably dead. Probably, but not certainly. In various circumstances, someone who appeared to be dead wasn't. Some drugs impede the respiratory drive, for example. And submersion in cold water can trigger a diver's reflex, which dramatically slows heart rate. For these kinds of reasons, physicians have long been called to the bedside to determine whether people have died—traditionally, not much of a diagnostic challenge.

Enter ventilator, stage left. A patient with massive brain trauma from a gunshot wound lies in an ICU, his heart beating normally. Without the ventilator, the patient would be dead, his brain so damaged he would have lacked the neurologic machinery to initiate a simple breath. A minute or two without spontaneous respiration and his heart would have stopped, leaving him dead by any of the most traditional definitions. But a dose of CPR and a breathing tube has kept his heart beating normally. Is he still alive?

The question seems to have an obvious answer—his heart is beating and his body is warm. But consider all those chickens running around the barnyard after having their heads cut off. Are they still alive?

The answer to this essentially philosophical question, of course, depends on what you mean by "alive." So let's try a simpler question. What is that chicken's prognosis? No matter how you define prognosis, the situation is grim. The only thing uncertain about this bird's future is whether it will end up in a stir-fry or a sandwich.

The Harvard committee was focused much more on prognostication than on philosophical discussion of what it means to be alive. They set out to determine what kind of brain injury would lead a person to have no chance of recovery. In fact, the title of the journal article laying out their criteria was not "A Definition of Death" but "A Definition of Irreversible Coma." They set out to establish the means by which physicians could determine whether a given patient, in a coma, had *any* chance of recovery. That the committee lacked data to support its claim of irreversibility, and that it focused on coma not death, did not stop the medical community from embracing the Harvard criteria as defining death itself.

What were these criteria? They included many measures of neurologic function: lack of brain stem reflexes, for instance, such as pupillary responses and involuntary withdrawal from painful stimuli. They included lack of spontaneous breathing and an isoelectric EEG reading, the latter reflecting a lack of electrical activity in the brain. The criteria necessarily included some judgment calls: three minutes off the ventilator with no attempt to breathe stood as proof of respiratory failure, not two minutes or four; isoelectric EEG readings separated by 24 hours, not 12 or 36. These judgment calls were necessary in order to be able to assess prognoses quickly enough that patients' organs would still be viable for transplantation, but not so quickly that the transplant teams would be procuring organs from patients who might otherwise recover.

I provide this brief overview of brain-death criteria in part because the lawyers fighting over Karen Ann Quinlan's fate entered into a lengthy debate about whether she was alive or dead. Karen's neurologist, Dr. Morse, spoke at great length in his testimony about the distinction between PVS and brain death, much of his discussion amounting to a courtside tutorial on brain science. Remember that PVS was a relatively new and mysterious diagnosis at that point, one that had only existed for a handful of years. Patients who would have died from acute brain damage only recently were now able to survive on ventilators, their acute injuries slowly resolving into chronic states. PVS so confused people at the time that one of the defense attorneys asked whether, if Karen was not brain dead, medical science could estimate her current "mental age." Was she equivalent to a two-week-old? A five-week-old? A seven-year-old? The best the neurologist could do was describe her as akin to an "anencephalic monster," a medical term for a baby born without any cerebral hemispheres. The Quinlans must have found this testimony quite disturbing.

All the technical talk about whether Karen was brain dead or simply brain damaged reinforced the authority of the physicians involved in her care. How could laypeople, even loving parents, be expected to make decisions for Karen if they couldn't even understand her neurologic condition?

A bunch of doctors had decided what counts as living or dead. They had talked about EEG readings and neurologic test results, all in enough medical detail that their criteria felt like a scientific judgment, even though their conclusion might have warranted a bit more input from philosophers and theologians. Senator Mondale had raised questions about the Harvard brain-death criteria in his 1968 hearings, but the world had responded with a shrug of its collective shoulders. Doctors make medical decisions, they thought, and the determination of death had always been a doctor's job. Why should that change now?

Their arguments made, the lawyers and family members awaited the verdict. They didn't wait long. In an opinion that rejected each and every one of Paul Armstrong's claims, Judge Muir concluded that New Jersey had "a compelling state interest in favor of preserving human life." To terminate Karen's treatment, he concluded, would amount to "homicide and an act of euthanasia."

The revolution had stalled, with doctors still ruling the day. In fact, as Muir put it, the decision to remove the ventilator was "inextricably involved with the nature of medical science and the role of the physician in our society and his duty to his patient." When it comes to life-and-death decisions like Karen's, he opined, "The conscience of our society places this responsibility in the hands of the physician."

Sorry, Mom and Dad. Doctor still knows best.

RISE OF THE ACTIVISTS

Three months before doctors discovered Betty Ford's breast cancer, Rose Kushner felt a tiny irregularity in her left breast. A confident career woman—a freelance medical journalist—Kushner did not rush to a doctor but instead headed off to her local library to conduct her own research *before* seeing any doctors. Had she gone straight to a physician, she no doubt would have been urged to see a surgeon immediately and cajoled into undergoing the kind of one-step procedure that the first lady went through later that fall: a biopsy under anesthesia, a quick look at frozen tissue under the microscope, and a radical mastectomy if the tissue looked cancerous.

Kushner was suspicious of the one-step procedure, however, because of concerns about the accuracy of the frozen section. With a frozen-section diagnosis, the pathology team takes tissue removed during the surgical operation and freezes it rapidly with liquid nitrogen. Under the microscope, this frozen tissue gives pathologists a pretty good idea of whether the patient has cancer. Pretty good, but not perfect. The more definitive pathologic diagnosis—called a permanent section—takes more time, thereby eliminating the possibility of a one-step procedure. Kushner did not think that the fate of a woman's breast should be left to the likes of a frozen-section diagnosis.

In fact, Kushner had encountered a morbid joke making the rounds at Johns Hopkins around that time that confirmed her view that no man would settle for a frozen-tissue diagnosis if his anatomy were at risk. As the joke goes, a medical student with a suspicious lesion on his penis undergoes a one-step procedure. Upon waking from anesthesia, he is told there is both good news and bad news.

"The bad news is that the frozen section showed cancer, so we had to amputate your penis," the doctor reports.

"And the good news?" the student wonders.

"The permanent section was benign."

Kushner was also skeptical of the need for radical mastectomy. Keep in mind that it was 1975, and the NCI trial confirming Kushner's skepticism hadn't yet been completed. But Kushner was a savvy enough reader of the medical literature to recognize a lack of evidence when she saw it. So instead of rushing off to see a surgical oncologist, she went to her primary care doctor. After much persuasion, she convinced him to perform a biopsy with no immediate plan for urgent surgery. He wasn't happy about being pushed around, but Kushner was nothing if not a force of nature.

When the biopsy revealed cancer, she went shopping for a surgeon who would perform a less invasive operation, a modified radical mastectomy. "She got eighteen straight rejections," according to medical historian Barron Lerner. But number nineteen was the charm!

After recovering from surgery, Kushner began her crusade so that other women wouldn't face the resistance she had faced. Linked tightly to the anti–Vietnam War effort, Kushner was a classic example of 1970s activism at its finest. An eloquent writer, she went public with her story, not mincing words about the misguided surgeons still promoting the unproven and unnecessarily disfiguring operation. Also active in the feminist movement, she wasn't shy about linking the radical mastectomy to the worst kind of sexist behavior either: "No man is going to make another man impotent while he's asleep without his permission. But there's no hesitation if it's a woman's breast."

The world needs activists like Kushner, unapologetic evangelists who won't shrink away from authority. Without near-fanatical AIDS activists, progress fighting that awful disease would have come much more slowly. Without protests, boycotts, rallies, and sit-ins, African Americans would have had to wait much longer to see civil rights gains. But sometimes progress is made as a result of more unlikely actors. As they say, it took a hard-line anticommunist like Nixon to improve relations with Maoist China. In a similar way, the case of Karen Ann Quinlan mesmerized the nation because it pitted a whole list of authority figures—the hospital, the doctors, the state prosecutor, even tradition itself—against an unassuming couple who had never seriously questioned authority in their lives.

Undaunted by Judge Muir's opinion, the Quinlans took their case to the New Jersey Supreme Court.

SUPREME JUSTICE

The Quinlans were not forced to sit once again through testimony about whether their daughter had the mental age of a seven-year-old. The New Jersey Supreme Court required only brief statements from the lawyers and a round of tough questioning. The justices asked and then seemed to quickly dismiss any question about whether Karen was brain dead. Was Armstrong "asking this court to change the common law definition of death"? Armstrong assured the court that he had no such intention. This was a case, he told them, about exercising the right of self-determination, not a case about the definition of brain death.

The justices continued probing Armstrong's intent. Was he "asking this court to order the doctors to do anything which they may feel contrary to their beliefs"? This was a critical question. For millennia, as we've seen, medical decisions were made by medical doctors. Were Armstrong and the Quinlans trying to upend all that tradition? Were doctors now to be beholden to patients, even if they disagreed with patients' choices?

"Absolutely not," replied Armstrong, appealing to tradition in order to bolster his argument. "We will do what is normally done in a physician–patient relationship. That is, if the doctor and the patient are at loggerheads, we would request that these particular physicians resign and ask to bring in another physician." Armstrong went on to lay out his view of how doctors and patients ought to work together to make medical decisions:

> The nature of the decision to be made by the physician is this, that he can give you a diagnosis; he can ask you as an individual what you wish to do with your body, especially in the circumstances where you are terminally ill and the treatment he advances is of no value to you. The physician can say, Mr. Jus-

tice, what would you do? Not, I'm going to employ this type of medical treatment regardless of what your particular views may be on the subject.

Armstrong must have assuaged the justices' concerns, because two months later the New Jersey Supreme Court handed down its unanimous decision. Joe Quinlan would be made Karen's guardian, and if he found a physician willing to withdraw her ventilator, that physician would not be legally responsible for killing Karen. If Karen's current medical team was unwilling to honor Joe's wishes, he was legally empowered to find her another physician.

The revolution had received its strongest push yet. The world had clung to the Quinlan story and had, consequently, learned for the first time about the amazing new technologies doctors could wield to keep their patients alive. But they'd also learned about these ventilators and feeding tubes and cardiac monitors at the same time they'd seen this equipment forced upon a girl and a family that wanted no part of these modern medical miracles. They'd heard the word "ventilator" linked with words like "forced." They'd witnessed two humble and loving parents brought to tears by physicians who acted as if no one else's opinion mattered.

I expect many people never looked at doctors in quite the same way after following Karen's story. Physicians are still held in high esteem by most patients in most parts of the world. Their advice is still valued and even sought out. But medical recommendations have never seemed so straightforwardly "medical" since the time of Karen Ann Quinlan. "You need chemo." Well, doesn't that depend on whether I want chemo? "You should have surgery." Hmm, doesn't that depend on my willingness to undergo short-term risk for long-term gain?

It has been almost forty years since the New Jersey Supreme Court ruled on the Quinlan case. In the rest of this book, I will paint a picture of where the revolution has left us. But first, back to New

Jersey, circa 1975. Karen was still on a ventilator and her parents had just learned that the State Supreme Court had accepted their point of view. Now it was time to return their daughter to a more natural state.

REVOLUTIONS DON'T ALWAYS HAPPEN OVERNIGHT

The story of Karen Ann Quinlan is not famous for being the first time doctors were forced to withdraw a ventilator from a living patient. No one was being forced to do anything here. If Morse was still uncomfortable withdrawing the ventilator, he could recuse himself from Karen's case, and the Quinlans could find a doctor more comfortable with their wishes.

The story is not even famous for being the first time a doctor voluntarily withdrew a ventilator from a living patient. Many of the journalists covering the Quinlan story had quoted medical experts who said such withdrawals were common. Many doctors, when faced with hopeless patients, told families that the ventilator was only prolonging the inevitable and the families went along with their recommendation to withdraw the ventilator. These decisions, however, were typically private. Most of the lay public hadn't known about such situations before Karen's predicament hit the media, but these tragic decisions hadn't been hidden. They had simply been made behind hospital curtains, between grieving families and caring physicians. Some of those curtain conversations had to have been bumpy. I expect that many physicians recommended removal of a loved one's ventilator only to discover that the family wasn't ready. In such cases, no doubt, the physicians continued offering intensive care to the patient, either until they died of other causes or the family changed its mind.

The Quinlan story was famous because the conversation had reached loggerheads and the family was pushing for extubation, not the physicians. It was famous as the first time a family, unable to agree with doctors about how to care for their loved one, chose to fight for their right to decide. And now that the court had answered the question of who had decision-making authority over Karen's future, it was time for the family to resume its conversation with Karen's physicians.

Julia telephoned Dr. Morse to set up a meeting. He seemed surprised that they wanted to see him, a reaction that struck Julia as unusual. She assumed that he had thought about how he would respond to the court's ruling. But instead, when they met, he acted as if nothing had happened. The Quinlans asked him what he planned to do in light of the supreme court decision. Morse said he hadn't read the decision, but that it wouldn't make a difference anyway—he planned on caring for Karen the way he'd always cared for her.

Joe somehow kept his emotions in check. "Does that mean you are going to ignore the supreme court? You're not going to do anything?"

Morse was unmoved. He explained that he was heading to Puerto Rico for two weeks, and didn't want anyone to make any rash decisions in his absence. "Be patient," he said while touching Julia patronizingly on the shoulder. "When I come back, we'll talk about it again."

It still pains me to think about what these wonderful parents were going through. Against all their natural inclinations, they had exposed the most horrific time of their lives to international scrutiny. They had stood up to a group of physicians whom they would have otherwise trusted with their own lives. And now, after everything they'd been through, nothing had changed?

Unbearable!

Worse than unbearable, in fact. Karen's doctors not only refused to withdraw her from the ventilator, they continued to add new technology to her bedside. When she developed a fever, they demanded a body temperature–control machine be brought to her room. New antibiotics found their way into her bloodstream too. In medical parlance, the doctors were still enacting a "full-court press" in an attempt to keep Karen alive. It looked like the Quinlans' only choice was to find a new physician and fire Morse and his colleagues from the case.

"No. Wait," the doctors protested one final time. They wanted one last chance to wean Karen from the ventilator. Not to extubate her, mind you. To *attempt* to do so.

"And if you take her off the respirator, and you find she isn't able to make it on her own, you will put her back on?"

Morse tersely responded, "I will."

"For how long will you continue to do that?"

"For as long as it takes," Morse responded. "Forever."

Nearly two months after the supreme court decision, Karen's doctors succeeded in weaning her from the ventilator. Weighing less than ninety pounds now, curled up tighter than a ball of yarn, Karen found the strength to breathe on her own.

She would live for another decade. She would receive antibiotics when her doctors felt she was getting pneumonia and tube feedings to sustain her minimal bodily function. But she would never go back on the ventilator. That, the Quinlans believed, would be playing God. And the Quinlans believed in leaving God in charge. They certainly weren't going to second-guess God's will. And by no means would they allow any physician to use extraordinary medical technology to stand in the way of God's plan.

They had finally wrested control of their daughter's care from the medical profession, and they had no plans to give it back.

PART II

Empowerment Failure

THREE

Lost in Translation

Katija Khisma had been admitted to the hospital because of a hard-hitting bacterial pneumonia, but the doctor was there to talk about her diabetes. Her blood sugars had fluctuated wildly in the first forty-eight hours of her hospital stay and he, the renowned endocrinologist, was there to get things under control. Seated at her bedside, he explained that the stabilization of her blood sugar was no small matter. "When your blood sugars rise too much," he said, "it interferes with your body's ability to fight the infection." Khisma nodded along. She knew how important it was to defeat this infection; her mother had died of pneumonia.

Encouraged by her nodding, the endocrinologist continued to elaborate on the importance of glucose control for her health. (Glucose is the more technical term for blood sugar.) He explained the relationship between insulin and glucose, describing how "the pancreas secretes insulin in response to rising levels of glucose after a meal, thereby helping move the sugar out of the bloodstream." Her nodding continued but with less assurance. Undaunted, the endocrinologist launched into an erudite soliloquy about white blood cell function and humoral immunity. (Or was it cellular immunity? Even as a medical resident observing this conversation, I often found myself struggling to keep up with his elaborate bedside pedagogies.) The patient kept nodding but mainly out of politeness; her eyes had glazed over somewhere between "immunomodulation" and "studies in mice have shown . . ."

I was becoming familiar with this look. It was the late 1980s, more than a decade into the patient-empowerment revolution, and I was training at the Mayo Clinic, a place that prided itself on giving priority to patients' needs and desires. Nestled in the not-so-bustling town of Rochester, Minnesota (itself planted in the middle of the only county I know of in the "Land of 10,000 Lakes" that has no lakes), the clinic recognized that the success of its business depended on satisfied customers, the kind who would rave enough to friends and family to convince them to fly to the wintry tundra.

That confused patient? I expect she was another satisfied customer. She certainly appreciated the time this kind and compassionate physician had spent educating her about her illness. He had made her feel as if he could spend all day talking with her, if she wanted.

The moral and legal battle over patient autonomy had largely been resolved by the time I reached the Mayo Clinic. By the late 1980s you would have had an almost impossible time finding a doctor in the United States who withheld cancer diagnoses from his patients. The practice of deciding for patients had also undergone a very dramatic shift. Studies of physician communication in the 1980s had revealed doctors deflecting patients' requests—questions like "What do you think I should do?" answered with "I can't decide for you" and "That is your decision to make, not mine."

The revolution had proceeded rapidly in the decade and a half following the Quinlan decision. Ethicists now wandered hospital corridors, called to bedsides by clinicians who had come to recognize that it was wrong to impose their own will upon reluctant patients. Physicians felled forests of trees to print out elaborate informed-consent documents that warned patients of even the most remote complications of their procedures. Researchers, too, had changed their ways. No more unwitting "volunteers." Ethics boards now reviewed research protocols in painstaking detail, their primary goals being to protect patients from unwarranted and unexplained risks.

Unfortunately, the revolution had proceeded at a pace exceeding doctors' and patients' abilities to keep up. Physicians were being told *what* they needed to do—inform patients about their medical alternatives and involve them in decisions—but were not trained *how* to do this effectively. Their moral duties had outstripped their communication skills. In trying to inform their patients about their health conditions, they were now confusing the daylights out of them. Motivated by the best of intentions, they were acting upon noble moral ideals of respect for patient autonomy and self-determination but frequently in such a clumsy manner that no one's best interests were served well. Doctors' well-meaning attempts to involve patients in medical decision making were too often lost in translation.

The patient-empowerment revolution is traditionally viewed by medical experts as a battle between laypeople and doctors over the right to make health-care decisions. Seen this way, the Quinlan case stands as an early and crucial victory for patient and family rights, a victory soon followed by many others. Throughout the '70s and '80s a series of lawsuits helped to strengthen the rights of patients and families to say no to medical interventions that their doctors were otherwise adamant about providing. Families won battles over withdrawing ventilators not only in patients with persistent vegetative state, like Karen Ann Quinlan, but also in alert patients with terrible diseases, such as ALS. They won the right to withdraw feeding tubes in terminally ill patients who didn't want their lives prolonged. The '70s and '80s were also a time of increasing regulation in medical research. Hospitals and medical centers now created institutional review boards (IRBs) to review research protocols and make sure patients and healthy volunteers were not unknowingly or unnecessarily being harmed by overzealous scientists. And, finally, it was a time when doctors became increasingly aware of their moral and legal duties to inform patients about their health-care alternatives, rather than leave them in the dark while deciding what treatment to offer them.

Seen from this perspective, as a power struggle between doctors and patients, the revolution has every appearance of being complete. The battles have been fought and the wars have been won. But the revolution should not be understood exclusively as a power struggle between doctors and patients. It should be seen as a struggle, undertaken by both doctors and patients, to work together to make good decisions. Surveys have shown that most patients reject the idea of being lone decision makers. They prefer to share in the decision with their doctors. Physicians, too, don't want to make every decision by themselves, without involving patients in deliberations. Orthopedic surgeons don't want to decide whether to replace anyone's hip without first talking to that person, to figure out whether they'll benefit from such an intervention. Most doctors and patients strive for partnership.

But to strive is not necessarily to achieve. The patient-empowerment revolution has failed because leaders of the revolution set a laudable goal out in front of doctors and patients—of partnering in making preference-sensitive decisions—without endowing either party with the tools necessary to lead to good decision making. Patients are too often unprepared for the shift in paradigms brought on by the revolution. Used to being underinformed and underinvolved, they suddenly find themselves under the care of physicians who have been taught about patient autonomy by those new bioethicists employed at their medical schools. The modern patient knows she is supposed to be a partner in her decisions, that she has a duty to get informed about her health and health care, but no one has taught her how to thrive in this new role. She knows she is supposed to act "empowered," but she doesn't feel ready to become the decision maker of last resort. Consequently, she finds herself dependent on her physician for assistance in living out the new paradigm.

And that's where things begin to unravel. As we'll see, the problem begins with the language of medicine, an arcane jargon that too often leaves the lips of clinicians who have forgotten that their words are not part of most people's vocabulary, only to land upon the ears of patients who either don't understand what their doctors are saying ("immunomodulation?") or think they understand without realizing that their doctor is using common words in uncommon ways.

BLIND TO JARGON

I coach youth basketball in my free time, and I pride myself on my ability to teach this complicated sport to kids who don't have much previous exposure to the game. Part of my talent as a coach is to identify when kids are struggling in a game situation and give them a quick way to improve their performance. Jacob keeps getting his passes intercepted? I pull him aside and remind him to fake his passes to see what the defense will do. Brilliant advice! Griffin keeps missing his fast-break layups? I show him how to jump-stop at the end of his drive so he can pull his shot together while the defense runs on by. Amazing? Not really. I simply know when Jacob and Griffin are panicking and give them simple techniques to slow down their play.

During one game, one of my players was getting burned on defense by a point guard who he was trying to cover all the way at half court. Standing at the sidelines, I tried to give Jorian the one piece of advice that would help him out. "Sag off," I told him. Jorian refused my advice, and his opponent dribbled right on by for a layup. I repeated my suggestion the next time we were on defense, a little more forcefully this time. "Sag off, Jorian. Sag off!" Soon, with Jorian still pressuring the point guard well above the three-point line, I was screaming louder than a Philadelphia Eagles fan. During the time-out I discovered that Jorian didn't know what I meant by the words "sag off."

Maybe I still have something to learn about coaching.

The more information that experts, like physicians, attempt to communicate to nonexperts, like patients, the greater the likelihood that some of this information will be wrapped up in incomprehensible jargon. For instance, I was supervising medical trainees in the hospital one month when I witnessed a conversation between a patient and a medical resident. The resident, who had graduated from medical school two and a half years earlier, was a better-than-average communicator and spent more time talking with patients than most of his peers, even sitting down at their bedsides to speak in slow, empathetic cadences calculated to soothe their anxieties. On the day in question, this resident was telling a patient that he might have leukemia.

"We are concerned," he told the patient in mellifluous tones, "because your peripheral smear showed some immature cells."

The patient responded with a befuddled stare, undoubtedly mystified as to what a peripheral smear was and puzzled about what kind of unruly cellular behavior would qualify as immature.

WHAT'S OLD WAS ONCE NEW

Medical school was tremendous for my vocabulary. Twelve years of Roman Catholic schooling and I had somehow avoided Latin, but once I began studying pathophysiology and anatomy, I found myself swimming in Latinate phrases: hypocellular versus hypercellular (the former means too few cells, the latter means too many), abduction versus adduction (the former means inward movement, the latter outward). In my first year of medical school, back in 1984, I drilled myself with flash cards, practicing long noun phrases until they felt like family names—chronic idiopathic pulmonary fibrosis, class III congestive heart failure, subacute bacterial endocarditis. The names just trip off the tongue, don't they? After learning these phrases, I began absorbing their abbreviations—medical language like CABG (pronounced "cabbage") for coronary artery bypass graft (also known as bypass surgery for the heart) and NSTEMI (pronounced "EnStemi") for a non-ST segment elevation myocardial infarction (a kind of heart attack).

Unfortunately, immersed as I was in medical lingo and surrounded for a hundred hours each week by my medical colleagues, I quickly forgot that these now-familiar words remained unfamiliar to most of my patients. A decade later, watching this medical resident toss out phrases like "peripheral smear," I had a vantage point that gave me easy access to the patient's state of mind. I wasn't thinking about what to say and how to say it, I was evaluating what the resident said and how he said it. My job, after all, was to make him a better physician. So I saw the confused look on the patient's face and stepped in to translate. But how many times earlier that week had I tossed off similarly meaningless mumbo jumbo to my own patients, too caught up in other matters to notice the befuddled looks on their faces?

Tape recordings have shown that doctors commonly use confusing jargon when talking with their patients, often without defining what their words mean. Even primary care physicians, who tend to focus much more on communication than specialists do, emit an average of five undefined technical terms per minute.

Many patients do not know that hemorrhage means bleed, that glucose means blood sugar, or that a suture is the same thing as a stitch. But most of us physicians have forgotten that we too didn't always know what these fancy words mean. I have asked countless patients with complaints of abdominal pain whether the pain hurts near their liver. But only recently did I learn that almost half of all patients believe their liver is located right above their pubic bones, where in fact the bladder resides. (The liver is actually located behind the lower right rib cage.) My ignorance undoubtedly interfered with my ability to communicate effectively with my patients. I would ask them questions using highfalutin medical words that I had mistakenly come to believe were lowfalutin ones. ("Does it hurt over your pancreas?") My patients, perhaps too embarrassed to admit that they don't understand what I am talking about, or maybe mistakenly believing that they do understand, answer my questions ("Uh yeah, it hurts right above my, uh, pancreas—yeah, my pancreas"), and we continue on, talking past each other.

To be fair, not all physicians are as clueless as I was about things like sutures and stitches. In fact, when I lived in Philadelphia, a wonderful little kid who lived across the street from me got banged up playing in his yard and was rushed to urgent care with a nasty head wound. Crying inconsolably, he asked whether the doctor was going to put a stitch in his head, a look of terror on his five-year-old face. And, as his mother tells the story, the doctor employed an absolutely brilliant use of medical jargon. "No, John," she said. "I won't use a stitch. I'll use a suture instead."

Hearing that, the boisterous boy breathed a sigh of relief. He came back to the neighborhood bragging that he hadn't gotten a stitch because the doctor "gave me a thooture," a story that sent our neighborhood into fits of laughter.

Unfortunately, such communicative intelligence is not the norm among us physicians. The world is full of great doctors and among them exist a subset of expert communicators. But these experts are definitely in the minority. Most of us physicians toss around medical jargon as if our patients are second-year medical students. And the consequences are frequently unfortunate.

Julian Samora, a communications researcher, tells a story about what almost happened to a patient named Amanda Jackson when she was in the hospital after giving birth to her first child. The morning after the delivery, the doctor walked into Jackson's room and asked if she had voided. She replied no, and the doctor left the room to find the patient's nurse to take care of her problem. A couple of minutes later, the nurse entered the room carrying scary-looking paraphernalia. Alarmed, Jackson asked the nurse, "What the devil are you going to do?"

"I'm going to catheterize you," the nurse responded, "since you haven't voided."

Jackson was familiar with the idea of catheterization and wasn't about to let this happen. "You're going to play hell," she said, realizing now, by the look of the catheter dangling in the nurse's hands, what the doctor had meant by "void." "I've peed every day since I've been here."

The nurse looked surprised. She thought the question had been asked and answered, not realizing that the patient didn't know the word "void" referred to urination.

The patient later explained the miscommunication. "Well, why didn't he just ask me if I'd peed? I'd have told him."

Good thing this woman was no shrinking violet. Many patients would not have been so lucky. In most of the tape-recorded studies I've reviewed, patients have listened passively while their doctors tossed off undefined jargon, rarely asking for clarification, even when they had no idea what the doctor was talking about.

Their passivity is not a coincidence. Doctors use jargon for many reasons, some conscious and some unconscious. But underlying all these reasons one looms large: jargon is a powerful way of establishing authority.

POWER TALK

Medical school found so many ways to make me feel stupid, despite the fact that I entered training with a surplus of intellectual confidence. A top student at my high school and an honors graduate of an elite college, I hadn't met many people I thought were smarter than me. But there is smart and then there is ignorant; medical school made me realize I was both.

At no time did I feel more ignorant than in my third year of training, when I began working in a hospital. All those clean, organized concepts crashed into the dirty, disorganized reality of patients whose diseases I had failed to study. Pneumonia masqueraded as heart failure. Migraine headaches fooled me into paging the stroke team. Here I was, crammed full of book smarts but painfully aware that I was an imposter, while my patients believed so wrongly that I was an expert, even while the short coat I was wearing screamed out to everyone else in the hospital that I was dangerously ignorant. (We medical students are typically the only people in the hospital whose lab coats halt above the waist.)

And then those first awkward encounters occurred, when I doled out to the patients indecipherable strings of jargon. I can't relay a specific story of one of these encounters, none of which landed with enough impact to register at the time. But I do remember the feelings I had when forced to translate for my patients, when they asked me what I meant, or probably more often when they looked so confused that I sat down to talk things through with them. In teaching hospitals, medical students often have more time to speak with patients than any other member of the medical team. And those conversations began to make me feel smart again. Drawing upon my book smarts, I realized how much more I knew about illness and disease than my patients. I almost began to feel like a doctor.

One of the ways we doctors entertain ourselves is with tales of medical lingo undergoing lay transmogrifications. The patient who refers to her women's health clinician as a "groinocologist." Priceless! The patient who told me he didn't want some "genetic medicine," which had me perplexed until he explained, "I want the trade-name drug instead." Aha—generic! Then there is the classic case of the woman who, when told she had fibroids in her uterus understood her doctor to have said that she had "fireballs in her Eucharist." Quite an image, when you think about it.

Jargon was key to my confidence—nothing like Latinate phrases to make me feel smart again. And with highfalutin jargon comes authority. Got a rash around your mouth? It would be disappointing if your dermatologist told you that you were suffering from "a rash around your mouth," and it would hardly justify the $500 bill. Doesn't "peri-oral dermatitis" sound better? Do you have high blood pressure for an unknown reason? Let's call it "idiopathic hypertension." Idiopathic is Greek for "I have no idea what the hell caused this."

I am in no way implying that medical jargon is designed primarily to impress or intimidate laypeople. Jargon allows doctors to commu-nicate to each other more precisely and efficiently. By creating new terms, physicians can use words that carry no additional meanings that could obscure the medical concepts being communicated. In addition, a good deal of medical jargon is a historical accident, car-ried down from the nineteenth century when scientists first started figuring out the root causes of disease. But jargon also creates space between professionals and laypeople. Indeed, patients have come to expect big words from their doctors. In one study, patients were asked to judge physicians who spoke in lay terms versus those who spoke in more technical language, comparing those who diagnosed them with an "upset stomach" versus "gastroenteritis," or a "sore throat" versus "tonsillitis." People understood the lay terms better, of course, but therein lies a problem. Anyone would have concluded that a patient with a sore throat has . . . a sore throat. Consequently, patients con-cluded that the doctors who used lay terms were less knowledgeable than the other doctors. They had less confidence in these physicians and were less satisfied with their medical care. Hard to blame physi-cians for speaking like physicians when that's what patients want!

The first barrier to shared decision making, then, is a language bar-rier, a gulf between doctors and patients created when physicians toss out arcane terminology, unaware that their words are not part of daily conversation, while their bewildered patients nod along "knowingly." But the linguistic confusion does not end with intimidating jargon. Even more dangerous are all those words doctors use that aren't so intimidating, the simple words that, unknown to most patients, take on more complex meanings in medical contexts.

SAME WORDS, DIFFERENT MEANINGS

George was nervous by nature, constantly fretting over every minor thing. If he thought someone had taken away the space he was about to park in, he would make a major scene out of it. He would obsess over whether his Frogger score was still the top one at the local arcade. So you can imagine how anxious he was waiting for the results of his skin biopsy. He had been concerned for a while about the white spot on his lip. Would it be cancer? Was he going to die?

Eager to resolve the uncertainty, he called his doctor's office for the pathology report. He was overwhelmed with grief when he learned the bad news. "My name is George Costanza. I'm calling for my test results . . . Negative? Oh my god. WHY! WHY! WHY? What? What? Negative is good? Oh yes, of course! How stupid of me."

The previous scene was, of course, fictional. But the *Seinfeld* writers had tapped into perhaps a bigger problem in medical communication than all of those Latin and Greek roots. After all, when a physician tells a patient he has polychondritis, the patient usually realizes that he has no idea what that word means. But when the doctor says "negative," but means it in a positive way—when doctors use common words in uncommon ways—there is a decent chance the patient thinks he understands what the doctor is saying even though he's mistakenly taking the doctor at his word.

I all too slowly became aware of this problem in my primary care clinic, when talking with hypertensive patients who weren't taking their blood pressure medicines as frequently as I had recommended. I would peruse a patient's pharmacy records and notice that he hadn't renewed his thirty-day supply of pills in more than sixty days, and I would toss off a reminder: "Now remember, Mr. Lee, you need to take your atenolol every day to keep your blood pressure in check." I might turn a computer monitor in his direction to show him that his blood pressure was rising. I would invariably hear excuses: "Well,

I got caught in bad traffic this morning and it has me anxious."

In the short run, anxiety from little things like traffic jams *can* raise blood pressure. Even the stress of having a nurse or doctor measure one's blood pressure can cause that pressure to rise, a phenomenon we in the profession call "white-coat hypertension." But many times I had seen evidence that the patient's elevated blood pressure was not transitory. So I would explain that, while this morning's blood pressure was artificially elevated because of bad traffic, he still had evidence of chronic high blood pressure on his physical exam or his EKG.

My education often failed to convince, because I had failed to remember that the word "pressure" meant something different to me than to my patients. To me, pressure was a concept from physics—the force of blood pushing against the arterial walls following cardiac contraction. To my patient, pressure was a feeling. You know, when you feel pressured, your blood pressure rises. After all, hadn't we just talked about this idea? Mr. Lee got caught in traffic, felt stressed out, and his pressure rose. Consequently, when he was home and feeling copacetic, why should he need to take a pressure pill? My problem was that I had assumed the patient used the word pressure the way I used it. A child of five would have understood this problem better than me, not having been immersed in the kind of medical training that takes common words and uses them in uncommon ways.

As Groucho Marx once said, send someone to fetch a child of five!

These kinds of miscommunications are serious problems, because they create a false sense of confidence in both doctors and patients that they understand each other. An oncologist tells a patient that the X-ray shows she had a "complete response" to chemotherapy. To a patient, that phrase sounds like "You're cured. The cancer is gone." But to a physician, that phrase means "There's no radiographic evidence of tumor," even in circumstances when the doctor knows the cancer is incurable and inevitably fatal. A pediatrician talks with concerned parents about whether their daughter has "an eating disorder" unaware that many laypeople think eating disorder is a synonym for "indigestion."

Simple words, eating and disorder, but not used in straightforward ways. Doctors are so used to the meanings their profession has grafted onto these words that they can no longer imagine why anyone would interpret their words any other way. The doctor has forgotten that the patient is not clued in to the special meaning of this phrase in this context.

One of the urologists I tape-recorded told a patient that his tumor, being early-stage, could be managed through watchful waiting. "What that means," he explained, "is we're not going to do anything and we're going to see if it [the cancer] changes at all."

What do you think the phrase "not going to do anything" means to a patient with newly diagnosed cancer? To the doctor it meant, "We will monitor the tumor carefully, watching for any signs of growth, ready to treat it more aggressively if it shows any signs of spreading." But to the patient it probably meant, "We're going to ignore it and hope it goes away." Would you be surprised to learn that this patient chose to have his prostate surgically removed?

Consider a family whose daughter had recently been diagnosed with Noonan syndrome, a genetic condition characterized by short stature and a varying range of physical and occasionally intellectual deficits. In her case, the symptoms were mild enough that the diagnosis was not made until after her tenth birthday.

The parents met with a genetic counselor, who went over the manifestations of Noonan syndrome with them in detail. Genetic counselors, it should be noted, rightly pride themselves on their communication skills. Helping people understand complicated conditions is a huge part of their job, and they receive more training on how to talk with patients than do the vast majority of physicians. Yet this couple came away from their meeting frightened and confused.

A researcher caught up with them at their house one week later, and they were obsessing over the word "syndrome."

"It frightens the life out of us," they explained, "because we don't understand it."

That simple word, syndrome, had thrown them into a tizzy because (and this all seems so obvious in retrospect) they were hearing it out of the mouth of a genetic counselor, and in this context it triggered a very powerful association.

"You think Down syndrome, and that's the only thing that sticks in your head, because you don't realize there are other syndromes out there. We were thinking she was a Down's, you know?"

I would never have thought they would think that. Down syndrome, really? A diagnosis so obvious it would never have been missed for ten weeks much less ten years. But what is obvious to us clinicians is obviously not obvious to the average parent.

For any pair of people to communicate effectively, it helps enormously if they share a common language. Unfortunately, as we have seen, doctors and patients too often believe they are speaking the same language even when they aren't, all the while clueless that the other party doesn't share their understanding of the conversation. These misunderstandings are all too human, reflecting our deep-seated bias to believe that other people are more like us than they really are.

FALSE CONSENSUS

Imagine you are a college student and have been approached by a research psychologist who hopes to recruit you into one of his studies, in which you will help him compare different kinds of persuasive language. To help him, you will walk around campus wearing a sandwich board that says EAT AT JOE'S. While wearing the sandwich board, you will keep track of who comes up to talk to you and what they say. Would you do it? It would be embarrassing, of course, but you would get course credit for your efforts and, more importantly, you'd advance science!

Okay. Now that you've made up your mind, estimate what percent of your peers, other students at your college, would agree to carry the sandwich board. When Lee Ross and his colleagues presented this scenario to Stanford undergraduates, they discovered that people's estimates of what *other* students would do were significantly biased by their own willingness to carry the sandwich board. Those students who said they would volunteer, for example, predicted that almost two-thirds of Stanford undergrads would also volunteer. On the other hand, those who weren't inclined to volunteer predicted that only one-third of Stanford students would do so. "If I find this embarrassing," they seemed to think, "so will others."

Psychologists call this phenomenon the false-consensus effect. Across a wide range of beliefs and behaviors, people assume that other people are more like them than they really are. The EAT AT JOE's example shows that people believe their behavior will be shared by most peers. Other examples show that people believe that their beliefs will also be shared by most of their peers. For example, Ross asked students if they thought there would be a woman on the U.S. Supreme Court within the next decade. (Ross conducted this study in the mid-1970s.) Once again, those who thought yes had assumed that two-thirds of their peers would also say yes, while those more pessimistic about women's chances assumed that only one-third of their peers would say yes.

Another phenomenon relevant to the gulf between doctors and patients is what psychologists call the spotlight effect. This phenomenon is nicely illustrated by a clever experiment led by Tom Gilovich, a social psychologist at Cornell University. In the study, Gilovich recruited half a dozen students and sat them around a table in a room in his lab. His research assistant then waited for a seventh student who was told upon arrival "to put on this T-shirt" before entering the room with the other students. The assistant handed over a shirt with a large head-and-neck portrait of Barry Manilow, a famous pop star who, at the time of the study—heck at probably any time in world history—was decidedly unpopular among college students. Then the research assistant took the unlucky seventh student into the room and directed him or her to sit in a chair facing the other students. Just as student seven was about to sit down, the research assistant interrupted: "On second thought, they're all too far ahead. Let's wait outside." The embarrassed seventh student then returned to the hallway, where one of Gilovich's other research assistants would ask, "How many of the people in the room you were just in would be able to tell me who is pictured on the front of your T-shirt?"

Put yourself in that student's shoes. You walked into the room late and obtrusively. Everyone looked up, wondering who you were, only to see you then walk back out of the room like some kind of lunatic. And to top things off, Barry Manilow's face was draped across your chest. If you are like most students who've gone through that experience, you will guess that at least half of those other people noticed who was on your T-shirt. But the actual number is closer to 20 percent. When we are embarrassed, the blood vessels dilate in our face, filling us with that warm, awful feeling of a blush, and we assume other people are acutely aware of our feelings. Often, those other people are too concerned about what we think of them to notice anything about us.

Here is a simple recipe for miscommunication. Start with a pinch of false consensus, a belief that other people will think what we think. As a consequence of this phenomenon, doctors talk to patients in a language patients don't understand, mistakenly assuming that patients will know what they're saying. Now add a dash of the spotlight effect, whereby the patient, feeling confused and embarrassed, mistakenly believes that the doctor must be noticing their confusion.

When the doctor then plows ahead, without clarifying his comments, the patient assumes the doctor doesn't care or that the information is not important enough to bother explaining.

Sigh . . .

ESCHEW OBFUSCATION

Most of the miscommunication I've described so far in this chapter is unintentional, with doctors trying their best to speak comprehensibly, all the while unaware that their patients are bewildered. On rare occasions, like the "thooture" story, miscommunication is not only intentional but wonderfully appropriate. Unfortunately, miscommunication sometimes serves more nefarious purposes.

In the mid-1990s, when I was a junior faculty member at the University of Pennsylvania, I had the good fortune to collaborate with a medical student, Ari, who felt that his student identity was being obscured by his superiors in an effort to encourage patients to let him practice procedures on them. Working in the hospital, the faculty would introduce him to patients as "Dr. Silver-Isenstadt," an outright lie that he would invariably correct, sometimes in the presence of the person who had purported the fib. More often, his identity as a student would be pushed into the background. No need to bring up that potentially unpleasant information.

Ari reached the breaking point when he spent a month at an affiliated private hospital that required its students to take off their Penn name tags, because the words "medical student" were displayed too prominently for patient comfort. To address this problem, Ari and I decided to conduct an empirical investigation of medical school name tags. We sent a letter to the deans of every medical school in the United States, asking them to photocopy an example of the name tag they required students to wear while working in the hospital. Unsurprisingly, most name tags were a simple variation of JANE DOE,

MEDICAL STUDENT. Others were more ambiguous: JANE DOE with nothing else. (In those hospitals, I guess the patients were supposed to realize that people in short white coats are students.) Yet other name tags were more creative: JANE DOE, STUDENT PHYSICIAN or JANE DOE, STUDENT DOCTOR. One name tag was quite concerning. In large letters it said JANE DOE, M.D., and then underneath, in half-size font, STUDENT.

We wondered how patients interpreted these various obfuscations. More specifically, we wondered how experienced they thought these students were compared to their superiors, to the "residents" and "interns" supervising them, words that we realized do nothing to indicate how experienced these people are as clinicians. Think about it. Why would someone who hasn't gone to medical school know the difference between an intern and a resident? And why would patients know that people with a label of INTERNAL MEDICINE HOUSE STAFF on their name tags (a synonym for a medical resident, someone who has graduated from medical school) would be more experienced than a STUDENT DOCTOR?

So we presented patients with a small pile of index cards labeled with these monikers and asked them to order the pile from least experienced to most. We discovered that most patients found these terms confusing. They often perceived "house staff" as being less experienced than the students they were supervising. No big words in the bunch—student, physician, resident, intern—but in this context, the meanings of these words were a mystery.

I think the medical school that designed a name tag with the word "student" in a minifont was purposely misleading patients so that they wouldn't worry about being cared for by neophytes. But I don't think most medical schools purposely mislead their patients. Instead, medical school administrators have simply forgotten that the words "resident" and "house staff" are incomprehensible jargon to an outsider.

I believe that most physicians spout jargon to their patients with no desire to confuse them. I think doctors are generally trying their best to communicate clearly to their patients, and such jargon simply feels like the clearest language. But we confuse our patients nonetheless. As a result of our jargon, patients often leave our offices in a state of "bewilderment unawares."

DISCHARGE INSTRUCTIONS

Carol Williamson had come to the emergency room with abdominal pain. The doctors had spoken with her, examined her tender belly, drawn blood, and even ordered X-rays. They gave her some medicine to reduce her pain, explained what they had found, and told her what she needed to do to continue her treatment.

Williamson told a research assistant that she was confident she had a thorough grasp of what had transpired in the two hours she had been under the care of the emergency room team. "What was the doctor's diagnosis?" the research assistant asked, as well as a series of other questions, pausing after each one to give the patient time to answer. Questions like, "What tests did you receive in the emergency department? What medicines are you supposed to take at home? Do you have any follow-up appointments? Is there anything you're supposed to watch out for?" The research assistant told the patient that she could refer to the discharge instructions the nurse had given her in order to answer any of these questions. Williamson did that, answering each question with unrelenting confidence. Sadly, most of her answers contradicted the hospital records. Her diagnosis? She'd thought they had found a stomach problem, but the doctors were actually concerned she had a sexually transmitted disease. Treatments? She thought she had received a shot of pain medicine, but she had actually been given an injection of antibiotics.

On rare occasions, we clinicians are such poor communicators that patients are forced to recognize our failures. Eric Cassell, a physician who has written two influential books on doctor–patient communication, recorded a particularly humorous example of this phenomenon: A physician had just told his patient that she needed to "have an EKG." The patient was puzzled by the medical term.

"A knee KG?" she asked. "My . . . my knee's okay. When it rains they hurt, but this is no trouble."

The doctor tried to clarify. "Uh, . . . no, it's connected to your heart."

"Huh?"

"You don't understand. An EKG is connected to your heart. That's why we do it."

"Knee KG?"

"You got it. That's what I'm saying." The physician was ready to move on to a new topic, his job as medical educator finished. The patient was ready to move on too, but not because the misunderstanding had been resolved.

She closed this part of the conversation with a shrug. "Knee in the heart? Uh, it's news to me. You're the doctor!"

I expect the physician had a good chuckle over that interaction. But all too often these misunderstandings are nothing to laugh at. Consider that woman who just left the emergency department completely unaware that she had been treated for a sexually transmitted disease. That is a dangerous bit of misunderstanding. How will she avoid a recurrent infection if she is unaware she was infected in the first place?

That woman participated in a study I conducted at two hospitals in Michigan with an emergency-medicine physician named Kirsten Engel. Engel and I were concerned that emergency room patients were being overwhelmed with information during their visits. They were interacting with nurses, lab techs, medical students, residents, staff physicians, and getting different parts of the story from each of these people but rarely getting a slow, careful explanation of what they most needed to understand about their acute problems.

So we hired a team of research assistants to interview patients as they were preparing to head home. We started off with low expectations, but we were still shocked to find out that only 20 percent of patients had a solid understanding of their emergency department visits, of what had happened in the E.R., and of what steps they needed to take to finish caring for their illness. And remember, each of them had a piece of paper in their hands providing them with information about many of the questions we asked. The problem was that they couldn't translate the discharge instructions into the concrete steps they needed to take to manage their health problems.

To make matters worse, most had no idea they were confused. When we asked them if they understood their diagnoses, they replied—almost universally—that they had a strong grasp of their situation. If patients had left the emergency department aware that they were confused, then at least they might have been motivated to ask more questions of the discharge nurse. If their doctors had told them *nothing* about their medical circumstances—if they hadn't even bothered to explain what tests they were ordering and what treatments they were prescribing—then at least patients would have *known* that they were in the dark.

One danger of the new paradigm is that physicians now explain so much so poorly to their patients, in an effort to involve them in their decisions, that patients often end up unaware of how truly bewildered they are. But that's just the beginning of the dangers. As I'll show in the next chapter, the miscommunications that plague so many conversations between doctors and patients are made all the worse by each party's inability to grasp what the other party is feeling.

FOUR

Blind to Each Other's Emotions

To prepare for our appointment, I opened up Joe Morneau's electronic medical record to see what other medical clinics he had attended since our last visit. I was disappointed to see that he had missed his appointment at the anxiety disorders clinic but was glad to see that he had shown up for his screening colonoscopy exam. Reading further, I saw that the gastroenterologist had removed several premalignant polyps—noncancerous growths that, if left alone, evolve into cancer over the course of many years. The gastroenterologist had also written a letter to Morneau informing him of these findings and had included a copy of that letter in the electronic medical record.

The letter was clear and concise. In the first paragraph it stated, "The results of your colonoscopy were" and then listed two options: "normal" and "abnormal." Next to the word "abnormal" was a box, filled in with an X. The second paragraph stated, "Your risk of colon cancer is," and then listed the options "increased" and "normal." The box next to "increased" was checked off. The final paragraph did not include check boxes but was a fill-in-the-blank statement, telling the patient, "You will be scheduled for another colonoscopy in _____ years," with the number "3" written in the blank.

I walked out to the waiting room to greet Mr. Morneau, who looked more anxious than usual. He and I made it less than ten yards down the hallway before he abruptly announced, "They told me I'm at high risk for cancer, but they aren't going to do anything about it for three years!"

On the surface, the letter was a paradigm of clear communication. It was made up entirely of simple, short sentences with nary a large vocabulary word (except for the term "colonoscopy," which it is fair to assume would be a term painfully familiar to him by then). The problem with this letter was not that it contained long words or unfamiliar jargon. The problem was that the doctor drafting the letter had forgotten what it feels like for a layperson to learn he has an increased risk of cancer. He hadn't succeeded in imagining how patients would emotionally respond to this message. In the doctor's mind, a polyp was (yawn) a benign little growth. He'd seen hundreds, maybe thousands of such polyps in his career. But many of the patients receiving this letter would be experiencing the first polyps of their lives, maybe their first brush with mortality. If not, then this would likely be the first serious thought they'd given to "the big C" in months.

To properly collaborate with patients in making difficult medical decisions, doctors need to not only communicate complicated information in ways that patients will comprehend but also anticipate the way patients are likely to respond to their words. When patients confront difficult medical decisions, it is counterproductive at best to be in the midst of an anxiety attack. In addition, when physicians interact with patients, they need to recognize and respond to patients' emotions. Unfortunately, physicians often fail to acknowledge these emotions—sometimes because they are clueless about what patients are feeling and other times because they don't know how to respond to those very basic human needs. Far too often what results is disaster: patients struggling not only with difficult decisions but also with strong emotions, and physicians forging ahead as if nothing is amiss. For the shared decision-making revolution to achieve its goals, both doctors and patients need to gain a better understanding of the psychological forces that blind them to each other's emotions.

PIVOTING OFF BAD NEWS

Four days earlier, Stanley Edgerton had lain down on his stomach while a urologist cut out twelve pieces of his prostate gland. He had sweated out the next few days, wondering what the biopsies would reveal. Now he was back in the urologist's office, ready for the news.

"The bad news," the urologist said, "is that, of those twelve biopsies, five of them did show some cancer in them, okay?"

"Ooh," Edgerton responded, clearly upset by the news.

"Now your cancer is a Gleason 6," he continued. "You have a normal DRE and your PSA is 4.58, so what that means is that you have a low-risk prostate cancer, and I'll tell you how many cores are positive as well."

"And what's . . . did you say DRE?"

"Digital rectal examination," the urologist explained. "So there are no nodules, but what your pathology shows is that—let me move this over [turning the computer monitor so the patient can see it]. What your pathology shows is that you have three cores that are positive for Gleason 6 prostate cancer and it's less than a 5 percent in each core, so it's not a lot of volume."

Where should I begin?

First, a bit of translation: The urologist was trying to reassure the patient. A Gleason 6 tumor is, actually, the earliest stage of prostate cancer. With no nodule palpable on the rectal examination and less than 5 percent tumor in the cores, the urologist is in the process of telling the patient that his cancer is about as harmless as a cancer can be. I expect that he's trying to stifle his patient's fears before they have time to flower. But rather than accomplish this worthy goal, he launches a jargon-laced diagnostic discussion that waylays the next five minutes of their conversation, in which the patient struggles to understand the difference between tumor stage ("At this point, you're T1 . . . I believe it's T1C because it's on both sides") and Gleason score ("You have . . . again, it's Gleason 6").

But I'm not relaying Edgerton's story to rehash the jargon problem I, um, hashed in the previous chapter. There is a second aspect of this story that merits our attention. In the midst of all his misguided efforts to educate this patient, and thereby calm him down, this urologist failed to perceive how his words would actually make the patient feel. The urologist *did* reassure his patient that his cancer was treatable: "It's in less than 5 percent of your cores, in three out of twelve, and basically what that means is that it's not a high volume and that it's low risk and that you have lots and lots of options to cure this, okay?"

But the patient is left to halfheartedly grunt "Uh-huh," perhaps confused about how three out of twelve something-or-others can translate into 5 percent.

I expect that most urologists recognize that their patients, upon learning they have prostate cancer—even early-stage, localized prostate cancer—are scared. But rather than acknowledge these emotions ("I know this must feel scary"), they try to convince them with rational scientific facts that they shouldn't be worried.

One of the urologists I recorded during my research had a clever turn of phrase he used in an effort to calm patients' fears. "Before we go any further," he told one man, "there are always two things I tell people. Number one, prostate cancer is a very slow-growing cancer. It's something people die with rather than of. It's not a death sentence."

That's a nice turn of phrase, "die with rather than of." But did the patient catch that clever elocution? It's hard to tell, because without any pause, the urologist continued:

"The second thing is that there are very good treatment options available for prostate cancer." The doctor then returned to the biopsy results and explained the patient's Gleason score.

There are many things I admire about this doctor's communication. Unlike many of the urologists we studied, he didn't launch into the Gleason score discussion without first taking a moment to reassure the patient that his cancer was not a death sentence. But still, he gave his patient almost no time to respond to the bad news, to react to the idea that he had cancer. I can see why the doctor doesn't want the patient to break down in tears before getting out the "die with rather than of" line. But must he launch into what would be an extended discussion of the Gleason score without taking a breath?

Imagine yourself in the patient's situation. You have just found out you have cancer, and the next phrase out of your doctor's mouth is "die with rather than of." Which word do you think will jump out of that sentence? "With"? "Of"?

My money is on "die."

When I teach medical students and residents how to deliver bad news to patients, I often refer to the Ginger syndrome, a phenomenon I named after a *Far Side* comic strip in which a pet owner, in the top panel of the strip, talks angrily to his dog Ginger: "Okay, Ginger! I've had it! You stay out of the garbage! Understand, Ginger? Stay out of the garbage!" In the bottom panel, we see the same words from Ginger's perspective: "Blah blah Ginger blah blah blah blah Ginger blah . . ."

I expect that this is how most people feel when told they have cancer, even a "mundane" one like localized prostate cancer. Overwhelmed by a shockwave of emotion, they don't hear "Your cancer is early-stage, a treatable cancer that has very little chance of reducing your lifespan . . ." Instead, they hear "Blah blah cancer blah blah blah cancer . . ."

In reading accounts of people's cancer stories, I regularly encounter the Ginger syndrome, even among people who epitomize the modern empowered patient. For instance, when Nancy Ainsworth-Vaughn, a sociologist with a Ph.D. in discourse analysis, learned she had cancer, she found herself overwhelmed by the verbiage her physician spouted at her. "After discussing with the surgeon at length what to do next, I drove home," she writes. "Then I tried to recount to my husband what had happened in the encounter. I could remember nothing about the discussion. All I could remember was that I probably had a malignancy."

Even medical professionals report being thrown into a state of confusion by their cancer diagnoses. Lawyer and bioethicist Carl Schneider quotes the response an experienced paramedic had upon receiving such a diagnosis: "I was in a bubble. I saw his mouth moving and I was aware of a flow of words, but I was unable to process most of the information. He might as well have been speaking a different language."

In the previous chapter we saw that doctors often *do* speak a different language than their patients. Now we see that, because they fail to recognize how bad news makes patients feel, their words remain foreign even to health professionals versed in the native tongue.

Shock. Fear. Bewilderment. It is normal to experience these emotions when your doctor drops a bad-news bomb on you. What people need in these situations above all is slow, compassionate time. I'm not talking about hours of therapy, even minutes of therapy; just a brief acknowledgment of feeling ("I know this must be shocking," followed by five or ten seconds of silence) or a recognition of the patient's state of mind ("I can see you're scared") can go a long way toward improving the conversation. A moment to let emotions begin to settle, then perhaps some calming words, when appropriate. Carefully chosen words, of course, not phrases centered on words like "die." How about something like "I know it feels awful to be told you have cancer, but you should know that your cancer is curable. We can treat this."

And then we doctors need to stop talking for a moment. The Gleason score can wait.

Patients should do what they can to slow down doctors too. Your doctor doesn't always know when you are freaked out. Trust me. I trained in Minnesota, where we cared for stoic northern farmers unparalleled in their ability to appear nonplussed by even the most shocking of events. If I had waited for the Ingmar Svensons under my care to show me, much less tell me, what they were feeling before treating their ailments, I'd still be in training. You, then, can do yourself and your doctor a favor by being explicit about your emotions. A study of patients with advanced cancer showed that when patients expressed emotion, half of the time they did so indirectly. This just increases the chance that the doctor is going to miss it and not address it. And when you face a critical decision and feel overwhelmed by your situation, by all means feel free to ask for a time-out. Most of us doctors will be grateful for knowing how you feel.

Not to suggest that we physicians will be experts in addressing your emotional needs. Strong negative emotions make all humans uncomfortable, even doctors who presumably encounter such emotions frequently in their work life. Indeed, one of the reasons your doctor may rush along your conversations is to minimize the odds that you'll bring up a painful subject. In my taped studies, I have noticed that most physicians hate silence. Consequently, many doctors offer patients time for reflection, but only for a brief and vanishing moment. "Do you have any questions," they will ask, followed by one or maybe two seconds of silence, a silence that makes physicians so uncomfortable they quickly move on to the next part of their agenda. A patient's only choice here is to either quickly come up with questions, overcoming the brain-freezing panic inherent to their situation, or make it clear—with gestures, if words aren't ready to flow—that they need time. Sadly, if patients don't exert some kind of control over these conversations, the majority of physicians will proceed, full steam ahead, unaware that the train is rushing down the tracks, its passenger still slack-jawed back at the station.

How did we physicians become so oblivious to the strong emotions brought out by illness?

WHEN DOCTORS USED TO BE LAYPEOPLE

The handsome young doctor tore the top off the packet with his gloved hand and removed the alcohol wipe. He rubbed it on the skin over his patient's vein, a vein now bulging because of the tourniquet he'd tied above her elbow. My wife, Paula, was already looking squeamish and the doctor hadn't even pulled out the—there it was, the syringe! Now Paula was wincing in anticipatory pain, the sense of pain only heightened by the fact that the mere sight of blood is enough to turn her stomach. The doctor plunged the syringe into her skin and drew the blood out in what looked like slow motion. Paula rolled away, pulling the bed linens with her, all the while pleading with me, "Tell me when it's over."

But she didn't have to wait long. The director quickly cut to a scene in another location. It was now safe for Paula to open her eyes and resume watching the television show. I chuckled at her reaction. Just seeing a television doctor pretending to draw blood from a television patient was enough to send her amygdala into overdrive. She looked my way, not pleased at my laughter, but good humored enough to laugh at herself. "I could never have been a doctor."

We physicians get that comment a lot. A child at the playground scrapes his head, a superficial wound but one with lots of bleeding, and whatever physician happens to be nearby is called into action, with people invariably amazed at how calm the doctor remains around so much blood. Dealing with death and dying, administering shots, cleaning out pustulant wounds—if it is sad, terrifying, or disgusting, doctors will handle it, surrounded by laypeople oohing and aahing over their ability to control their emotions in the face of such unpleasant circumstances.

In my high school freshman biology class, my teacher showed us a movie of a woman giving birth. Partway through the delivery, one of the smartest students in our class, Tom Schreier, excused himself from the room to sit in the hallway, his skin pale even by Minnesota-in-February standards. He decided that day he was not going to be a doctor.

I almost joined Tom in the hallway, my own future in medicine in great doubt. Here's the secret: Most of us physicians used to be just as easily shocked, scared, and grossed out as anyone else. It was only by repeated exposure to sick patients—literal exposure to their blood and guts—that we got used to the sights and smells of illness. Medical training is a long process of emotional desensitization.

Such desensitization is essential. If we doctors never got used to the sight of blood or pus, we couldn't do our jobs. But that doesn't mean, as medical students, that our stomachs didn't turn the first dozen times we had to clean an infected wound. If we physicians experienced prolonged sadness whenever one of our patients died, none of us would be able to practice as oncologists, geriatricians, or intensive care specialists. But that doesn't mean we weren't distraught as medical students the first time a patient died under our care. It doesn't mean we don't feel upset later in our careers when our patients suffer and die. It still hurts, but it doesn't hurt quite as much or quite as long. It can't or we wouldn't be able to practice medicine. Becoming desensitized is a slow process, one that isn't the result of conscious effort, just emotions that slowly diminish over time.

Sometimes desensitization is sped forward by humor, deeply inappropriate **medical** humor. Thinking back on my time as a medical student, I remember how distressed I felt interacting with severely demented patients, their mouths wide open, vacant looks on their faces. I also remember the shock of hearing the medical resident who was supervising me make a joke about one such patient as he signed out to the night float team. The sign-out is an important medical ritual, during which one physician describes his patients to another so that the latter physician can take care of those patients overnight. On that evening, my resident began telling his colleague about one of his patients, a demented woman he described as having "a positive O-sign." Responding to my befuddled look, the resident clued me in on the strange jargon. " 'O' when they're like this," he said imitating the openmouthed look on the poor woman's face, "and 'Q' when they're like this," now repeating his imitation but this time sticking his tongue out of the corner of his open mouth. The other resident softly chuckled—not at the "joke," which he had no doubt heard many times before, but at the sight of another innocent medical student furrowing his brow at the dark discourse of doctorly desensitization. I was disturbed that day, but that didn't keep me from repeating this line of humor the first time I could relay it to someone even less desensitized than me.

People under stress often cope by resorting to gallows humor. Freud recognized this coping mechanism, writing in 1927 that the ego responds to distressing situations with humor to show that "such traumas are no more than occasions for it to gain pleasure." Psychologists much more recently than Freud have demonstrated that humor builds social bonds among people who are working together in stressful situations. When sociologists have studied the working relationships of physicians and residents in a hospital, humor has jumped out as an important way that not only helps physicians separate themselves from others—nurses, patients, and hospital staff with different concerns—but also enables them to bond with each other and cope with common problems. But for all its purported benefits, the desensitizing effects of gallows humor, and of medical training more generally, creates enormous problems for doctor–patient communication, leading to interactions in which patients feel strong emotions and their doctors don't. Just as importantly, this desensitization can cause doctors to lose the ability to see the world through their patients' eyes . . . even when those eyes are closed, as I learned in my third year of medical school in a crowded O.R.

A "HARMLESS" EXAM?

It was 1987 and I was halfway through my month of OB-GYN rotation, one of the required rotations for us third-year students. I gloved
my hands and walked into the operating room where the head surgeon, upon seeing me, got all excited. "Student, get over here," she
barked. "You need to examine this woman before we start the operation. You'll never get a better chance to feel pelvic anatomy."

I glanced around the O.R. and what felt like a sea of eyes stared
at me impatiently—the anesthesiologist, the nurses, the OB-GYN
resident—all wondering when I would get moving so they could proceed with the operation. I approached the patient and began nervously
palpating her abdomen. I inserted two fingers from my right hand
into her vagina while gently pressing down on her abdomen with
my left hand, her uterus and ovaries now palpable between my two
hands. Anesthesia had paralyzed the woman's muscles; consequently,
when I performed a pelvic examination on her, she didn't tighten her
belly like she would have if she had been awake. I could almost begin
to make out the shape of her uterus. It would take several similar examinations before the anatomy started making sense to me.

I had performed something that all medical students need to perform: I had practiced my exam skills on a patient so that, one day, I
could master that skill. But I had *not* done something equally crucial
that day. I hadn't asked that woman for permission to practice upon
her anesthetized body, and neither had the surgeon.

How could the surgeon and I have thought that it was acceptable
for me to probe this woman's most private parts without her knowledge? I can only speak for myself. To begin with, I was frantically
obsessed with learning my new trade, meaning that each clinical encounter was a precious opportunity to practice my skills. In addition,
I wanted to impress my superiors and get good grades. So when I
stood there in the O.R. that day, presumably facing a moral dilemma,

I barely gave the situation a second thought. The little feeling of moral uncertainty that rose in my chest? I squelched it with tortured logic. The surgeon, I reasoned, was a wonderful person, passionately dedicated to medical education. So if she thought it was okay for me to examine this woman, then it must be okay. Besides, I told myself, I am a medical professional; there was nothing prurient about my behavior.

In my research, I have asked women how they would feel if they learned that medical students were practicing pelvic exams on them without their permission, and most have said they'd be horrified; they'd feel violated. Yet when I've asked doctors about this topic, I've usually received a very different response. It would be nice, they say, to ask permission before conducting such exams, but it often wouldn't be feasible. It might even cause undue worry among patients. "Is it really appropriate," one doctor asked me, "to increase their anxiety by consenting them to a harmless pelvic examination?" (consenting being the word doctors use to indicate that a patient has given them consent to do something).

In the mid-1990s, I studied this issue with Ari Silver-Isenstadt (the person I collaborated with on the name tag study) and we discovered a disturbing fact. The further students progressed in their medical training, the less important they thought it was to ask permission before practicing sensitive portions of the physical examination on their patients. Attitudes toward the specific practice of performing pelvic examinations on anesthetized women shifted dramatically when students rotated through the OB-GYN service. Most students entered the rotation with a natural instinct to find this practice un-ethical, but after seeing good physicians perform unconsented exami-nations, after being put in the awkward position of conducting such examinations themselves, it no longer seemed awful. Psychologists would probably file this under "cognitive dissonance"—when people feel the pain of contradiction, they usually find some way consciously or unconsciously to reconcile their contradictory beliefs.

Medical training, having desensitized doctors to a wide array of situations, creates an empathy gap between doctors and patients. At the same time, it causes doctors to forget how they used to feel before the extraordinary became ordinary.

Barron Lerner recounts an extreme version of this desensitization in his book *The Breast Cancer Wars*. A surgeon stands with his patient in the center of a medical amphitheater. The year is 1963, and the surgeon is extolling the virtues of the radical mastectomy operation that he had performed on the patient just weeks prior. A member of the audience raises his hand. "Did the patient have feelings about losing her breasts?" the student asks. The surgeon's answer reveals that the patient's opinion is irrelevant, even if it were her feelings that were the focus of the question. Missing breasts, he says, have "no cosmetic value." The patient sits, silent. No one asks for her thoughts.

Shocking, absolutely shocking. I'm tempted to say the behavior is inexcusable. But I'm not here to pass moral judgment on that surgeon. I'm trying to give you a better idea of how medical training and medical practice lead to empathy gaps. The surgeon that day was so focused on his theory of cancer treatment—that removing more tissue increases the chance of a cure—that he couldn't imagine a patient having different priorities. That surgeon probably felt strong emotions the first time he violated the integrity of a patient's skin with a scalpel. He probably felt a twinge of unease the first time he cut away healthy muscle to get to the underlying pathology. It had to have been hard for him to look at the chest of the first woman who received a radical mastectomy under his care. But now, having performed dozens of similar procedures, the operation no longer caused him to feel strong emotions. When he pulled off her gown to expose her missing breasts, all he saw was a postoperative specimen. In his mind, this woman had nothing to be embarrassed about. But from her standpoint, she must have been mortified. He had lost sight of her feelings.

Keep that surgeon in mind the next time you talk with a physician about an emotionally painful topic. I bet my upper molars that your physician will be more sensitive than the surgeon was that day. For starters, that was 1963, and for all I've said about current physicians and our frequent failure to anticipate patient emotions, I expect we fail less often than our predecessors, who were trained in the patient-as-guinea-pig era. Nevertheless, that surgeon acts as a reminder to all of us that physicians, despite good intentions, may not realize when their patients are embarrassed.

NOT PREPARED FOR PATIENTS' EMOTIONS

Scott Mackler is one of the smartest physicians I have ever met. He combines great analytical skills with an almost freakish memory and an ability to absorb new facts—to file them away within his preexisting "hard drive"—all in a manner that still allows him to see the big picture. As I imagine Scott's brain architecture, I envision separate neuronal pathways for facts about, say, pneumonia and heart failure, cross-referenced for areas of overlap (when congestive heart failure presents as pneumonia), replete with open spaces to add new information: "Interesting article in this week's *JAMA*; I'll have to file that under pneumonia, antibiotics, and randomized trials."

So when Scott developed ominous neurologic symptoms, his brain quickly formulated a thorough differential diagnosis—doctor talk for a list of diseases that could potentially cause these symptoms. The muscles in Scott's right forearm were firing spontaneously, in a pattern that he immediately recognized as an early sign of amyotrophic lateral sclerosis (ALS), a disease better known in the United States as Lou Gehrig's disease. Only a little more than forty years old at the time, with two energetic teenage boys at home, Scott racked his brain for alternative diagnoses, *anything* to avoid that most dreaded of diseases—an illness that, if he were really suffering from it, would in a matter of months or years strip him of every ounce of strength in his body, leaving him wheelchair-bound and dependent on a ventilator to breathe, if he even chose to go on a ventilator.

Scott went to see a neurologist, hoping the doctor had heard of some disease, any disease other than ALS, that could explain his symptoms. But the neurologist did not give Scott any new diagnoses to cling to that day. He didn't give him any old diagnoses either. In fact, the neurologist refused to even acknowledge that Scott's symptoms were consistent with ALS.

Scott was taken aback by this lack of communication. Visibly upset, he pushed the doctor for details. But the neurologist refused, saying it was too early to speculate. Too early to speculate? Didn't this neurologist realize that Scott was already speculating? That horse had sprinted out of the barn already. Scott just wanted to know where it might be heading. Scott had come into that appointment with some informational needs. He had wanted a differential diagnosis and an idea of how they would proceed with testing. But because of his medical background, Scott's informational needs were minuscule compared to his emotional needs. What Scott really needed that day was for someone to acknowledge his awful situation.

As we've seen, the medical profession has a long and ignoble tradition of withholding diagnoses from patients, out of fear that patients won't be able to handle the truth. But that tradition was not what Scott encountered that day. There was no ALS diagnosis to withhold from Scott. The neurologist was correct to tell Scott that he needed more time and tests to reach a definitive diagnosis. So the neurologist wasn't technically withholding a diagnosis from Scott but simply withholding a list of *possible* diagnoses. To what end? To keep Scott from experiencing undue alarm? It had to have been obvious that Scott was already deep in very due alarm. Yet somehow the neurologist was oblivious to Scott's emotional needs.

Clinical encounters are often emotional affairs. Unfortunately, far too often the emotions spill forth from worried patients only to be ignored by their physicians. James Tulsky and Kath (pronounced "Kat") Pollak, medical communication experts at Duke University, have conducted a series of groundbreaking studies on how physicians do (or

more often do not) respond to empathic opportunities when interacting with patients.

What exactly is an empathic opportunity? Tulsky and Pollak are
quite conservative in identifying such opportunities, only counting
the moments when patients audibly express feelings of negative emotion. A furrowed brow or a worried look doesn't qualify as an empathic opportunity by their definition because their research involves
tape-recording, and such facial expressions are invisible to their audio
recorders. By contrast, a sigh or crying or a pained utterance—"I'm
frightened"—would count as an empathic opportunity, an unambigu-
ous emotional cue that physicians have a chance to respond to. Consider the following conversation from their collection, one that took
place between an oncologist, a patient, and the patient's friend.

The friend discusses what a shock it was to learn that the cancer
had come back with a vengeance. "You guys [referring to the patient
and the patient's husband] had talked about starting a family. The
timing was so unfortunate because we really all thought—the doctor
had thought, everyone thought—we had it beaten. It's done. Just to
have it come back, so sudden and so fierce."

"Then out of the blue I started having back pain," the patient adds.

"It was doubly hard," said her friend. "You had all these great ad-
ditions to your life. Everything was going so well. It was doubly hard
the second time."

The oncologist finally joins the conversation. "Do you have sib-
lings?" he asks.

In this interaction we hear a clear emotion followed by a clear
nonresponse to that emotion—a patient and her friend pleading for
compassion and receiving no help, nothing in return.

Such responses are all too common in medical practice. For every
doctor who responds empathically to a patient's expression of negative
emotion ("I can imagine how scary this must be for you"), two shut
the door on any kind of emotional talk ("Let me just interrupt. What

we are seeing is lymph nodes . . ."). Patients express powerful fears in explicit terms ("I worry about my kids having no mother") and even though doctors have no choice but to recognize these emotions, many still find ways to push the emotions into the background: "Yeah, it's not easy. But before we talk about that, let's talk about your appetite."

How could we doctors be so callous as to brush off the suffering? In part, it is the result of all that desensitization I wrote about earlier. Perhaps we don't see any reason for the patient to be so scared, so we dismiss their emotion. I'm all too familiar with this response. Once I asked one of my research managers to evaluate how well I was running my research center, and after interviewing my employees, she reported to me that several of them were upset about my tendency to dismiss their ideas with a characteristic hand gesture and change of topic.

Ouch! It is never fun to learn you are acting like an ass. I realized, once I got past denying my behavior, that I often entered research meetings having given the topic at hand more thought than my research assistants who, after all, weren't fifteen years into their research careers. Thus, when they would present legitimately good ideas, but ideas that I had already studied before or had thought through, I wouldn't acknowledge the value of their ideas but would push the conversation ahead with a dismissive wave, making them feel ignored and unappreciated.

Since being alerted to this tendency, I have tried to pay attention to this behavior, so I can correct it. I even began noticing similar behavior in my clinical practice. The umpteenth patient would come to my office, worried about what I considered to be an insignificant situation, and I would find myself wanting to move beyond this mundane issue to something more important. But it didn't matter that I wasn't worried about the situation; what mattered was that my patient was scared. I was missing out on empathic opportunities because I had become desensitized to the kinds of "old and boring" health problems afflicting my patients, problems that were neither old nor boring to them.

But desensitization to emotions is not the only reason physicians miss out on empathic opportunities. In some instances, I expect physicians are all too aware of their patients' emotions, and in response experience strong emotions themselves, unpleasant feelings that they don't know how to handle. When I went to medical school in the mid-1980s, for instance, I was given almost no training on how to respond to patients' emotions. As a result, I have since found myself responding to patient "complaints" (the inelegant term we physicians use to describe any mention patients make of feeling less than well) with a sinking feeling of my own, one part compassion-fatigue and another part inadequacy. Because I can't think of any way to reduce the patient's suffering, I become uncomfortable discussing their complaint.

A patient complains of pain, telling me that my previous efforts haven't cured his illness, and I feel upset, maybe even defensive. So rather than acknowledging my patient's emotions ("I know you are frustrated") or putting voice to my own emotions ("I feel bad that I haven't been able to help you more"), I pivot the conversation away from such feelings to land on more comfortable terrain ("Well, let's see if that new pill is affecting your kidney function").

Assisting me in my pivoting, turning my pivot into a virtual pirouette, is the new paradigm of patient empowerment. The paradigm isn't based on emotion but on cold hard logic. Lawyers argue their cases in front of judges. Lawyers team up with philosophers to convince medical schools that patients have an ethical right to be involved in their decisions. It's hard to think of two professions more logical than law and philosophy.

And we physicians, trained under this new paradigm, have become understandably obsessed with information. Our patients need to get up to speed on as many medical facts as possible if they hope to share in the decision at hand. No time, then, for emotions.

What a shift from the day of Hippocrates. Back then, remember, physicians concerned themselves almost exclusively with patients' emotions, having nothing else to offer them. Then the scientific revolution struck, and physicians busied themselves curing patients, even experimenting on them without their knowledge. Now, with the new paradigm, doctors are starting to communicate more with their patients, often inelegantly and incoherently, as we saw in the previous chapter, but at least they are putting forth an effort. The same cannot always be said for the way we physicians respond to patients' emotions. Our duty to inform patients has turned into a crutch with which we hobble away from those unpleasant feelings intruding on our medical deliberations.

WHERE MATTERS STAND

The patient-empowerment revolution has been fueled by logic and reason. It was started in part by lawyers, arguing in front of judges and juries about the legal basis for the right of patient self-determination. It was further fueled by ethicists, who filled medical journals with arguments extolling the moral primacy of autonomy and found the time to jam Kant and Mill into crowded medical curricula.

But where will all this logic lead us if we don't attend to emotion? In my bioethics training, I learned a great deal about moral argumentation. I imbibed scores of articles praising the virtues of giving patients a bigger role in their health-care decisions. I don't remember ever being told that it was important to recognize my patient's emotions, or to train myself to acknowledge these emotions, or even to develop awareness of my own emotions. In my medical training, my professors drilled me repeatedly on how to interpret subtle EKG findings, and on how to analyze acid–base disturbances based on urine and serum electrolytes. But no professor ever taught me what to do when my patients tell me they are frightened.

Patient advocates are similarly uneducated about the role that emotions play in modern medical practice. I've read several popular books on patient empowerment, inspiring tomes that encourage laypeople to take hold of their medical problems, educate themselves about their illnesses, and stand up to their physicians should they encounter doctors who aren't otherwise inclined to involve them in their care. Rarely mentioned in these books are the issues that have surfaced in this chapter.

If you strive for empowerment—better yet, if you strive for partnership with your physician, a topic I'll address in parts III and IV—keep in mind the likelihood that both of you are underappreciative of the other party's emotions. Good decision making requires good communication. And it is hard for two people to communicate effectively with each other if they don't understand how the other person feels.

FIVE

Misimagining the Unimaginable

He could make the trip from bed to bathroom with his eyes closed, having hurried over that path more nights than not since being diagnosed with ulcerative colitis ten years ago. He couldn't remember, in fact, the last time he had made it through the night without that rushing, rumbling feeling. Daytime was miserable too—especially the cramping, a pain that would double him over like a Swiss Army knife returning to its owner's pocket.

Experts don't know what causes ulcerative colitis, whether antibodies get revved up on their own or whether they are spurred to action by a bacterial invader (and the colon is loaded with bacteria, forcing the immune system to make thousands upon thousands of decisions about which antigens to ignore and which to attack). Whatever the explanation, the consequence was clear. Edward Hollingsworth's immune system was treating the lining of his colon like an uninvited guest. His main symptoms were bloody diarrhea and intense cramping pain, in addition to what doctors call tenesmus, a kind of sphincteric false alarm involving a rush to the bathroom with nothing to show for it. He had these symptoms despite being on maximal medical therapy, including pills to suppress his immune system and suppositories to reduce inflammation. The medicines had prevented him from needing emergent hospitalization, but staying out of the hospital was not the same as living a symptom-free life.

So when he came to my clinic for his annual physical, I decided to talk with him about how to get his colitis under better control. I brought up the one treatment he was still not in the mood to discuss. "If you want to rid yourself of your colitis," I reminded him, "maybe we should talk again about surgery."

Ulcerative colitis can be a nightmare of a disease, but even at its most horrifying, it is limited to the victim's colon. Hence, if a patient is willing to part with his colon, through a surgical procedure called a colectomy, he will essentially be cured of the illness. No mucosal cells for the immune system to attack anymore, no more need for prednisone or mesalamine or any of those other nasty medicines. No more colon, though, meaning Hollingsworth would have to live at least for a while with a colostomy—his bowels, rather than snaking through his belly to his anus, would now be interrupted five or six feet short of their normal destination, forced to expel their contents through a hole on the side of his abdomen into a removable plastic pouch pasted to his skin. That's right, he'd have an open hole a few inches above his belt buckle; he would poop into a plastic pouch.

He could not bear the thought. "Oh God, no. I would be miserable with a colostomy."

"But aren't you miserable already?" I asked him. He shook his head no, vigorously. He assured me life wasn't all that difficult, certainly not difficult enough to contemplate a . . . he wouldn't even say the word. He assured me that he would rather stick with the devil he knew.

Did he make the right decision? Was he correct to predict that life with a colostomy would be worse than his current battle with ulcerative colitis? In the previous two chapters, I painted a picture of some of the problems that have plagued doctor–patient communication since the dawn of the patient-empowerment revolution. Modern physicians try earnestly to explain health-care facts to their patients, aware now that patients deserve a role in medical decision making.

All the while, neither party is fully aware of when such explanations are adequate and whether such explanations should leave patients reassured or anxious.

But even when patients comprehend the choices they face, they may make decisions they will come to regret. Because people like me, who study behavioral economics and decision psychology, know that both patients and physicians are prey to unconscious forces that could lead them astray. In the next few chapters, I'll explore some of these forces, starting with the phenomenon that influenced Hollingsworth—a frequent inability to accurately predict the long-term emotional consequences of unfamiliar circumstances. Later in the book, I'll lay out some things we all can do to improve our decisions.

THE DECISION TREE

As we have seen, the new paradigm of patient empowerment was promoted by two rigorously logical professions: law and philosophy. Each had a certain credibility that held sway with doctors. Bioethicists drew upon two thousand years of philosophical thinking in arguing for the importance of patient autonomy. Any physician who struggled through Kant in an undergrad philosophy course had to have *some* respect for the bioethicists now nestled in the medical education building. Lawyers had perhaps even more credibility among physicians than bioethicists; after all, they had convinced the courts that doctors have a legal duty to inform patients about their treatment alternatives, meaning that doctors had to acknowledge this new paradigm or risk their medical licenses.

But not all physicians found these prophets of the new paradigm to be entirely credible. Many found bioethicists to be a bit otherworldly, too abstract, and yes, too philosophical for their liking. And lawyers . . . well, doctors had no choice but to follow the letter of the law; nevertheless, they did not have to like doing so. When doctors failed to inform patients about their treatment alternatives, it was malpractice lawyers who took them to court, a branch of the legal profession regarded with disdain by most physicians. To be fully persuaded of the value of the new paradigm, physicians needed to hear from a more credible source. They needed to be exposed to a more clinically and scientifically grounded line of argument.

Along came the field of decision analysis. Decision analysis is a discipline that grew out of the intersection of economics and mathematics. Its experts take complex decisions and statistically model them on what are called decision trees, to point decision makers toward the best alternatives in cases too rich with options for the best alternative to be otherwise apparent.

Consider a very simple decision: whether to accept a $10.00 prize now or take a chance, based on the flip of a coin, at winning $25.00. Heads you win, tails you lose. This decision can be represented with the decision tree below:

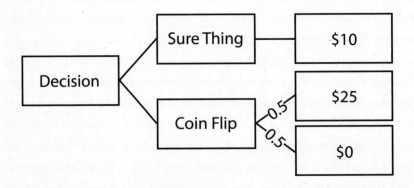

This decision is too simple to require decision analysis, but it nevertheless illustrates how this powerful technique works. The decision tree above shows the two choices. With simple math, we can calculate the *expected value* of each choice. For the sure thing, we know that we can expect $10.00 at a probability of 1 (where zero equals no chance and 1 is a sure thing). Thus, the expected value is:

$$1 \times \$10.00 = \$10.00$$

For the barely more complicated coin flip, we face two possible outcomes, each with a probability of 0.5 (50 percent chance). The expected value of the coin flip therefore is:

$$(0.5 \times \$25.00) + (0.5 \times \$0.00) = \$12.50$$

Of course, no one who chooses the coin flip will win $12.50. They will either win $25.00 or go home empty-handed. But the expected value here represents the *average* outcome. When making a decision many times, or when making the same decision for many people, the average is a pretty important outcome. If one medical treatment yields an average life expectancy of, say, ten years and another yields one of twelve and a half years, that information would be important in deciding which treatment should become the standard of care.

To grasp the power of decision analysis, imagine a more complicated decision. Let's say that one alternative involves risky cardiac surgery. The surgery carries some chance of curing the patient's symptoms, some chance of doing no good for the patient, some risk of minor harm, and a low risk of death. Among those who improve with the surgery, a proportion will develop further heart disease down the road while others will develop other diseases. These probabilities stack up on earlier probabilities; some outcomes, like surgical complications, occur early and others occur later in the treatment course. A decision analyst builds a branch for each of these health outcomes, even adding in fancy "time-release" branches (things like Markov nodes—don't worry about the technicalities!) to better capture the range of possible futures facing patients who choose this alternative.

Oh yeah, and the analyst goes through the same tree-building process for each alternative. If, as an alternative to surgery, the patient can receive a stent—a wired tube designed to prop open a cardiac artery from the inside—then the decision analyst will have to build a tree analyzing every likely consequence of a stenting procedure. The coin flip pictured above illustrates a decision tree with only three branches. A decision tree for a complicated situation would contain dozens of branches, the tree alone filling up a couple of pages of a medical journal in a font size readable only by those thirty-five years or younger. Pretty impressive stuff. Very scientific. The kind of rigorous logic that even a skeptical physician can admire.

But what does this have to do with the new paradigm? Let's return to our simple coin flip, a sure $10.00 versus a fifty-fifty chance of $25.00. What should you choose?

Suppose you are the world's most rational person and you face this choice dozens of times. You would be wise to take the coin flip every time, because it has a higher expected value. But suppose you faced this decision only once; in this case, the right choice is not so obvious. Maybe you want to go to a movie tonight and you need $10.00. Lose on the coin flip and your evening plans are ruined. It makes sense, in that circumstance, to go for the sure thing. Now suppose instead that you hope to ask someone out to the movies tonight and can only do so if you win $25.00. In that case, $10.00 has almost no value to you. Better take a shot at the coin flip.

The right choice, then, depends on how much you *care* about each of the outcomes—in this case, it depends on what you think you would feel and experience if you had zero, $10.00, or $25.00. Decision analysis experts call the value that a person places on an outcome—how much they care about each outcome—utility, a word they borrowed from economics (after it borrowed the same word from moral philosophy). If, in your present circumstances, you have a strong preference for $25.00 over $10.00, you will opt for the coin flip. If your preference is weak enough, you won't take the chance of ending up with nothing.

Decision analysts have developed ways to quantify these preferences, or utilities, to point decision makers toward the right decision.

And this is where we return to the new paradigm. Because the utility of any given medical outcome—like the utility of $10.00 versus $25.00—is a matter of individual preference.

Consider a man choosing among prostate cancer treatments. A group of decision analysts draws out a decision tree, each of its branches representing a potential treatment outcome. One branch might end at "surgical wound infection," another at "severe incontinence." Resting on each branch is a probability estimate, a piece of data culled from the medical literature indicating the likelihood each health outcome will occur. At the end of each branch, hanging like an October apple, is the utility that each patient places on the outcome in question. Enter the preferences of a patient who places a low utility on incontinence—in other words, someone who truly hates the idea of living with incontinence—and the decision tree points eagerly toward watchful waiting. That patient's best interests are best served by avoiding that particular side effect. Enter the preferences of a patient who instead places a low utility on living with untreated cancer inside his body, and the decision tree will point toward a more aggressive treatment.

What the decision analysts proved, with their impressive mathematical models, was that patient preferences mattered—that the "right" decision was not purely a medical matter but depended on combining medical data (the probabilities of all the relevant medical outcomes) with patients' unique preferences. Many physicians, especially those steeped in the new science of evidence-based medicine, found this argument convincing. Hard-core research types, academic physicians who believed in data and science, found decision trees more compelling than philosophical references to Kant and Mill.

But those of us trained in behavioral economics aren't so thoroughly enamored with an analyst's decision trees. Logically speaking, we recognize that decision analysis is useful in showing people what they ought to decide. But what if the preferences, the utility values, inserted into the trees are flawed? Or, to translate that last bit of gobbledygook into English, what if people's preferences are screwed up because they don't know what it's like to experience the outcomes—incontinence, colostomies, etc.—relevant to their decision? Do patients really know what they want? Are the preferences they express for various health conditions really the kind of preferences we want determining medical choices?

EATING GROUND GLASS

Good medical decision making often depends on patients being able to accurately imagine what life will be like if they make one choice versus another. A man with localized prostate cancer, for example, must guess whether he will be unhappier with impotence and incontinence after surgery or with the anxiety accompanying active surveillance, knowing that an untreated cancer is living within his body. A patient with chronically infected leg ulcers has to guess whether he'll feel better continuing to fight the ulcers and their accompanying pain or receiving a below-the-knee amputation. One alternative—the devil he knows—over the other—so permanent, so drastic, so unimaginably horrible. But would it really be so bad to lose the bottom of his leg?

As it turns out, people frequently misimagine their own long-term emotional reactions to unfamiliar circumstances. Consider some important nonmedical decisions: A man moves to Southern California, convinced that the sunny weather will more than make up for the cost of living, all the while unaware that most people receive only a temporary boost from the new climate. He emotionally adapts to good weather, taking it for granted before he's made it through his second winter.

A woman purchases a lottery ticket convinced that a big win will bring her long-lasting happiness. But the thrill of the victory soon abates, competing for emotional salience and attention with the unforeseen consequences of new riches: old "friends" who hit her up for cash, an early retirement that leaves her wondering how to spend her time. A round of golf was so much more special when those four-hour blocks of time were scarce.

I have observed this type of misimagining among faculty colleagues over tenure decisions, as if any remaining chance of happiness depends on the committee's recommendation. The junior faculty members I've spoken with predict, almost universally, that they'll be miserable if they fail to receive tenure—not just miserable that month or over the next year while they scramble for a new job but deeply, permanently miserable, as in life as they know it will be over. They are wrong, very wrong. People have an impressive ability to bounce back from a wide range of adversities. Those rejected for tenure usually find other universities willing to hire them, sometimes schools a rung or two down in the academic hierarchy, but schools with really smart and interesting faculty colleagues and with young students who ask great questions.

Dan Gilbert and Tim Wilson, two of our era's finest social psychologists, call this underestimation of emotional resilience "immune neglect." People, they argue metaphorically, have psychological immune systems—an array of emotional defense mechanisms that kick in whenever they feel bad. Those grapes? Probably sour. That gubernatorial candidate you hated who won the election? Maybe he's more moderate than you thought.

When bad things happen people feel bad for a while, so they look for ways to feel better. But prior to those bad events, when imagining how such circumstances will affect their lives, people systematically underestimate the speed and strength of this so-called psychological immune system. When they think about how they will feel if their football team loses the big bowl game, they imagine days, maybe weeks, of sadness. Yet usually within a matter of hours they have distracted themselves with other thoughts. When they imagine their long-term response to tenure rejection, they think about the shame they will feel and about the burden of moving to a new city. They fret over what it will be like to work at a less prestigious university. All the while, they neglect the likelihood that their self-esteem will remain intact: "Can I help it that I value teaching more than my peers do?" And they overlook the odds that moving to a new city will be exciting.

Immune neglect is a common phenomenon in health-care settings. Ed Hollingsworth was a victim of immune neglect when he imagined that life with a colostomy would be miserable. In my research, when I have measured the quality of life of people with colostomies, they have reported the same moods and similar levels of life satisfaction as people who don't have colostomies. The same kind of immune neglect exists for a whole range of medical conditions. For instance, my colleagues and I measured the moment-to-moment moods of dialysis patients over the course of a typical week. These patients were seriously ill, facing an average annual mortality rate of 20 percent, yet we discovered that they were in positive moods the vast majority of their waking hours. In fact, when we compared their moods to those of a "control group"—healthy people matched to each dialysis patient by age, race, education, and gender—we could not find any difference. Patients with end-stage kidney failure—tethered to dialysis machines ten-plus hours per week, a few bananas away from life-threatening potassium levels—were happy just as often as their healthy peers.

I don't mean to suggest that people are impervious to circumstance or can bounce back from any type of adversity like a punch-me clown. Some adversities overwhelm even the most resilient of people. And some people are overwhelmed by relatively modest challenges. But, in general, people underestimate their emotional resilience. The power of emotional resilience is often astonishing. This power is a great benefit to humankind, allowing us to bounce back from a wide range of adversities. But this surprising resilience can wreak havoc on medical decision making. If people underestimate their emotional resilience—if they misimagine the unimaginable—they might make bad choices.

An old saying asserts, "He who lives by the crystal ball soon learns to eat ground glass." How can patients avoid making bad predictions?

WHAT DO THEY KNOW?

When Ed Hollingsworth recoiled at the idea of a colostomy, I had not yet done research on how colostomies affect people's quality of life. Even so, I had already developed a sneaking suspicion that most people with colostomies thrive despite their condition. And Hollingsworth, in my view, would have probably felt better with a colostomy than he felt with his uncontrolled symptoms. So rather than take his decision as final, I pushed back, asking him to collect some data for himself.

"When do you have your next appointment in the GI clinic?" I asked.

"Next month," he replied.

"Why don't you talk to some of the other patients there, maybe even see if the nurses will introduce you to people who have colostomies. Then you can ask them what it's like."

A few months later, I saw Hollingsworth again and asked if he had followed my advice. He had, he told me, and the patients reported that living with a colostomy wasn't nearly as bad as they had thought it would be. It was far better, in fact, than living with the symptoms of ulcerative colitis. But he continued to resist the operation. "They told me they were happy," he said, "but I simply can't believe it."

Why is emotional resilience so hard to fathom?

BEFORE I GET OLD

In the fall of 2010, I hiked the foothills of the Swiss Alps with my friend Amalio Telenti—two middle-aged physicians contemplating the onset of old age. I was forty-eight at the time and Amalio was a touch older. We were both as fit as we had ever been in our lives, ready to outrun or outhike most men half our age. Our wives, too, were middle-aged but still the objects of younger men's desires (at least in our minds). We felt we were on top of the world. But for how long?

"This isn't going to last much longer," Amalio mused. "Another decade, maybe two, and we will be old, undeniably old. Our best years," he sighed, "will be behind us."

It had been a pretty exhilarating hike up until that time. But now I felt myself peering not up toward the snowcapped peaks but forward in time to a future filled with decline—graying hair, further decaying of my joints, a man no longer able to kid myself that I was still a kid.

In 1965, the British rock group the Who released a song that *Rolling Stone* magazine would later call the eleventh greatest rock song of all time. "My Generation" reached number 2 on the charts in the United Kingdom (only number 74, though, in the United States—what's wrong with Americans?), with Roger Daltrey stuttering through Pete Townshend's provocative lyrics. "I hope I die before I get old," one line rang out, a lyric Townshend reportedly penned in anger at England's Queen Mother, who had told the local authorities to tow Townshend's car, a hearse she found to be an eyesore. Easy for a rocker in his twenties to look at a cranky old blue-haired woman and believe that death would be a better fate than to reach such an age. Easy for a healthy forty-eight-year-old hiking the Swiss Alps to ponder his future and conclude that it's all downhill from here.

But I knew better. I had seen the data with my own eyes. I'd even collected some of it, research proving that happiness and well-being don't decline with age but instead typically increase. Surveys have consistently shown that the average seventy-year-old is happier than the average thirty-year-old.

I bring up the topic of happiness and aging for two reasons. First, I want to reinforce my theme of misimaginings. Pete Townshend wrote that he would rather die than get old; at the time I wrote this book, he was thriving well into his seventh decade. He was wrong about his future, as are most young people. The thirty-year-olds I have surveyed predict a significant decline in happiness over their lifespan, a prediction strikingly at odds with the data. They do not foresee happiness as older people because they don't realize that with age comes a certain amount of emotional wisdom, an ability to brush off negative experiences more quickly than they were able to do in their youth.

In fact, when researchers at Stanford University exposed people to a series of video images and tested people's memories, they found that older people were just as good at remembering the positive images as the younger people, but significantly worse at remembering the negative images. In effect, they were editing out emotionally unpleasant experiences as they encountered them. To people who doubt this phenomenon, I suggest spending ten minutes (max!) with any MTV reality series. See how well twenty-somethings handle disappointment and cope with social rejection, for instance. The smallest slight and many twenty-year-olds spend days in a tizzy. Older folks are better at avoiding these negative experiences. For starters, they stop spending time with people who get on their nerves. But even more importantly, when they are slighted or when they experience other adverse circumstances, they are better at letting such negative feelings roll off their backs.

Unfamiliar with the wisdom that comes with age, the typical thirty-year-old assumes that seventy- and eighty-year-olds are unhappy. Who can blame them? Twenty- and thirty-year-olds, when pondering old age, think about wrinkles and dentures. Do they contemplate people like my hero, Jack LaLanne, who lived well into his nineties and could toss off dozens of finger push-ups and brag that he "still has sex almost every day—almost Monday, almost Tuesday, almost Wednesday . . ."

Which brings me to the second reason I'm exploring age and happiness: to report to you that older people have no better insights than younger people do about how happiness changes over a lifespan. As I mentioned, in my research I discovered that the typical thirty-year-old mistakenly believes that happiness declines with age. Somewhat surprisingly, the majority of seventy-year-olds believe the exact same thing. Despite experiencing the wisdom that comes with age, they believe themselves to be less happy now than they were in their youth. They misremember what it was like to be a young adult. Reflecting back on their youth, they remember flexible joints and the exhilaration of falling in love. However, they seem to forget the negative emotions they experienced as thirty-year-olds—the uncertainty about career and family, for example, or the struggles they faced over their finances, or the stress they experienced due to existential doubts.

Older people misremember the happiness and unhappiness of their youth because their beliefs about aging and happiness—that younger people must be happier—contaminate their memories. If you want to ask people how an experience has changed their lives, then you can't necessarily trust them to give good answers. This has important implications for medical decision making. People facing difficult medical decisions commonly seek out patients who have been through related experiences, hoping to gain insights from them, much like Hollingsworth did when I referred him back to the GI clinic. Will the patients unwittingly give them inaccurate forecasts? Consider my study of dialysis patients, whose moment-to-moment moods were indistinguishable from their healthy peers. I asked these patients, after they recorded their own moods for a week, to tell me what they think their moods would have been like if they had never experienced kidney failure. They imagined a level of positive mood that was significantly greater than what healthy people actually experience.

Ask a dialysis patient what her life is like and you will probably hear "I'm happy" or "I'm doing okay." But dig a little deeper, asking them how their kidney failure has influenced their moment-to-moment moods, and they will say something like, "Well, I'm happy now, but I'd be a heck of a lot happier if I wasn't so sick."

Clearly life is better with functioning kidneys than without, but dialysis patients are wrong to think that having healthy kidneys will be reflected in their moment-to-moment moods. They don't realize that their psychological immune systems have purged them of the negative emotions associated with their health problems. Kidney failure is awful, but people rarely feel awful about their kidney problems for very long.

If you cannot get accurate information about how a specific illness changes people's lives from patients—the people who've experienced the illness—can you at least get better information from doctors? Unfortunately, you can't. According to a host of studies, doctors are even more clueless about how illness affects people's lives than patients. For example, researchers surveyed women with breast cancer and assessed their quality of life across a whole bunch of life domains: their overall quality of life, their ability to function in social environments, and the like. They also asked close relatives to gauge the patients on each of these same domains, with the idea that relatives would have insight into when patients were, say, holed up in their bedrooms avoiding social contact. And the data backed this up. Patients and relatives were generally on the same page in reporting the patient's quality of life.

Physicians, on the other hand, weren't even in the same chapter. Across the board, they underestimated patients' quality of life. They were even less conscious of people's ability to emotionally adapt than were the patients themselves.

Now, I recognize that concepts like "quality of life" are vague and, therefore, ratings of quality of life can be wigglier than a fresh bowl of Jell-O. Nevertheless, large disparities in perceptions of illness still occur between patients and physicians, even when the perceptions aren't limited to Jell-O-like topics such as quality of life. For example, when researchers surveyed married men with prostate cancer, they confirmed that patients and their spouses were generally on the same page when it came to reporting how the patient's life was going. When asked whether the patient—the man—was still interested in sex, husband and wife gave usually identical answers, which when you think about it makes sense. They were also on the same page when describing how frequently the patient was having night sweats.

By contrast, physicians were often way off in estimating how patients were faring. They overestimated patients' interest in sex, for example, as well as their appetite, how often they had night sweats, and even the amount of pain they were experiencing. In addition, they underestimated how close patients felt to their spouses. There was only one issue in which doctors and spouses agreed with each other while parting ways with patients: Doctors and spouses overestimated how important the patient felt it was to have erections.

The moral of this story is sadly straightforward. If you have an important medical decision to make and need information on how a specific health condition might affect your life—on how it will feel to have an amputation, say—don't expect your doctor to know.

So whom can you trust? My best advice is to trust other patients, as long as you ask them the right questions. Ask a patient "How has your amputation affected your life?" and you're treading on dangerous ground. They'll probably misremember their pre-amputation life and thereby overestimate the impact the amputation has had on their current life. It's better to simply ask them questions about how they're doing right now. "Are you happy?" isn't a bad place to start. Better yet, get specific. "Can you walk up stairs okay? Does phantom limb pain keep you awake at night? How often do you have pain from your prosthesis?" People are generally good at answering these kinds of concrete questions about their current life. It's when you ask them to make broad judgments about now versus then that they go astray.

And finally, when you ask them these concrete questions, you'd do well to believe their answers. When the colostomy patient says he's happy and almost never feels that other people notice his device, his answer is the best estimate you're going to get about how a colostomy will affect your life.

When people make medical decisions, they contemplate unfamiliar and often disturbing circumstances: hair loss from chemotherapy, incontinence from surgery. In contemplating these possible outcomes and in choosing treatments that will minimize the chances of these outcomes, they could very well be making mistakes. If you misimagine the unimaginable, you might choose an option that will make you worse off.

SIX

Beyond the Numbers

We discussed how his new medication would benefit both his blood pressure and his heart. He nodded as if he agreed with the importance of taking the pill. But then a worried look came over Jorge Hernandez's face. "Any side effects?" he asked. I explained that most patients had no problems at all with this medication, although some had dizziness for the first few days and a few had a cough that went away with discontinuation of the pill. "Yes, but could it cause serious side effects?" Almost every pill could do that, I replied. But for this pill, any such side effects are extremely rare.

"Like what?" he asked. "What kind of side effects?"

I was hit by a sinking feeling, one I expect most clinicians have felt in their career. I was doing my best to educate this patient about his treatment alternatives, describing common side effects without scaring him about extremely rare complications, ones that I had not seen more than a few times in my career. Nevertheless, this looked like a losing battle. "Well," I continued calmly, "on very rare occasions people can get kidney problems."

"Serious ones?"

"Well, Mr. Hernandez, most people just get a bump in their blood test that almost always goes away when we stop the pill."

"*Almost always?*" Our conversation continued for a while more, but the end was already in sight. He would not be taking this pill any time soon.

As I explained in the previous chapter, the new paradigm of patient empowerment was given a strong intellectual boost by the relatively new discipline of decision analysis, a field with trees full of probabilities and utilities that sort out difficult decisions at the same time as they demonstrate the central importance of patient preferences in determining which decision is "best." These decision trees lay out the logic of decision making—of how people *ought* to decide—taking rational account of likelihoods. For example, all else equal, a rare outcome should play a smaller role in determining a person's best choice than a frequent outcome.

Yet here I was talking to a man who seemed obsessed with tiny probabilities, with the remotest of risks. But risks that I felt compelled to inform him about. Earlier in my career I had worked on an institutional review board (IRB), a committee that exists in research hospitals to protect the rights of potential research participants, making sure no one is subjected to experiments without knowing the likely risks and benefits of their participation. Due in large part to entities like IRBs, researchers no longer waltz into modern-day Willowbrooks and inject unsuspecting people with hepatitis virus or cancer cells. (Hurrah!) Also due to IRBs, researchers rarely enroll people in research studies without first introducing them to a list of the potential risks of their participation, including those risks that are quite remote. My experience on the IRB had shown me that enforcers of the new paradigm—my fellow IRB members—were adamant about providing patients with information about even the remotest possible risks of research protocols before they would allow patients to participate in studies.

But my IRB experience, as well as interactions I've had with patients like Mr. Hernandez, has caused me to reflect on the new paradigm. I know patients deserve this kind of information, so they can decide if the risks associated with their pills are too great to warrant taking the pills. But I am not sure whether laying out all these risks for patients is promoting rational decision making. I don't know how much information to give my patients, whether a list of rare side effects, for example, will simply scare them away from what is in their best interests.

Scratching my head one day after one of these disturbing clinical encounters, I decided it was time to run an experiment. The experiment involved a hypothetical situation. I asked people—in this case, laypeople eating lunch in a hospital cafeteria—to imagine they had been diagnosed with colon cancer and that there were two surgical procedures that could potentially cure them of this cancer.

To get a feel for my experiment, let's pretend for a moment that you are one of those people diagnosed with colon cancer. Here is what we know about your two treatment options:

The first surgery, the *uncomplicated surgery,* has an 80 percent chance of curing you of the colon cancer without any major surgical complications. There is, however, a 20 percent chance it won't remove all of the tumor and you will die as a result of the cancer.

The second surgery, the *complicated surgery,* has a better chance of curing your cancer, but at the cost of several rare treatment complications. Like the first surgery, it has an 80 percent chance of curing you without any major complications. But there is a 16 percent chance it won't cure you and you will die of the cancer. What about the missing 4 percent? That's the odds that you will be cured—you won't die of the cancer—but you will also experience a surgical complication: a 1 percent chance you'll be cured but have to live with a permanent colostomy, a 1 percent chance you'll be cured but have chronic diarrhea that gets you out of bed one night per week to race to the bathroom, a 1 percent chance you'll be cured but experience a surgical wound infection that takes up to a year to heal, and a 1 percent chance you'll be cured but have scar tissue in your belly that causes occasional abdominal pain.

To be clear, no one with colon cancer faces a choice between these two operations. I made up these treatments and treatment outcomes in order to see what people would choose—specifically, to find out whether a short list of relatively rare complications would scare people away from what otherwise looked like the best choice. After all, these treatment complications, as bad as they might be, can't hold a candle to death. This choice really becomes one of "give me colostomy or give me death."

The vast majority of people I have surveyed say that, given a choice between death and permanent colostomy, they'll take the colostomy. They say the same for the other treatment complications. As bad as it is to experience any of these complications, it would be even worse to die. That means the best choice for most people will be the complicated surgery, which gives them a 4 percent better chance of surviving their cancer.

But that's not what most people do. When faced with this hypothetical choice, the majority of people choose the uncomplicated surgery. I have asked many people about their reasoning. One typical conversation went something like this:

"What would you prefer, death from colon cancer or permanent colostomy?"

"The colostomy."

"Okay. Death or diarrhea? Death or a wound infection . . ."

"They are all better than death."

"Okay then, if you had to choose between surgery 1 and 2 [I never called them the "complicated" and "uncomplicated" surgeries on the survey], which one would you pick?"

"I'd pick surgery 1, the one without the treatment complications."

With a befuddled look overtaking my face, I asked, "Didn't you just tell me that those complications were better than death from colon cancer?"

"Yes, I did. But I just can't bring myself to pick that operation. Something just doesn't feel right about it."

This simple little experiment highlights the tension lurking below the surface of our shiny new medical paradigm. Many of us doctors have learned through experience that when we leave patients to their own devices—even after we've armed them with comprehensible information to make their decisions—they often behave in ways that appear irrational. Saying you prefer colostomy to death, for example, and then choosing a treatment with a higher death rate just to avoid complications like colostomy, is inconsistent at best. It suggests that some strong irrational impulse is preventing patients from choosing the option that best fits their own preferences.

Most doctors recognize that medical decisions are no longer purely medical affairs. We have swallowed the lessons spooned into our mouths by lawyers, ethicists, and decision analysts—that values are a crucial part of determining what is best for any given patient. And while not all doctors have mastered clear communication, we also know that clarity alone will not make patients into good decision makers. Take this little colon cancer experiment, for example. People understood the information I provided them. They stated clear preferences: colostomy is better than death, diarrhea is better than death. Yet when it came down to making a choice, they couldn't pull the trigger on what they knew was the best decision.

Good decision making is not merely a matter of comprehension. Understanding doesn't necessarily lead people toward making rational choices. Decision making is often as much about feeling as it is about thinking. And the way people use risk information, such as statistics about how likely they will be to experience side effects, is often influenced less by their understanding of the magnitude of these risks than by subtle psychological cues that change the way these risks feel.

NUMBER CRUNCHED

When confronted with the strange way in which patients factor risks into their decisions, most experts lay the blame on misunderstanding. They attribute patients' odd behaviors to confusion over the facts. If patients don't understand the risk information relevant to the decisions, the experts contend, how can we expect them to make rational decisions?

There is plenty of reason to be concerned about how well patients understand the "statistics" relevant to their decisions. Not surprisingly, given the glimpses of doctor–patient communication laid out a couple of chapters ago, patients are often confused about the facts because doctors frequently present these facts to them in a confusing blur of verbiage. For example, in a tape-recorded encounter an earnestly communicative hematologist described the risks and benefits of treating leukemia to his patient, trying to explain that there is a good chance that her tumor will respond to chemotherapy: "So, if you look at complete cytogenetic response rates in the chronic phase, it's about 80 percent, and if you look at the accelerated phase, it's about 15 percent. So the drug doesn't work in advanced disease very well. If you look at patients who get a complete cytogenetic response as their best response in the IRIS trial, their risk of ever progressing in the next four years, so about forty-eight months roughly, is about 8 percent overall."

"That's good," the patient replied.

"Yeah. And this is divided into people who become Philadelphia chromosome positive but appear to be in chronic phase. And half of these are people who go to accelerated phase or blast crisis. If you look at people who had complete cytogenetic response—this is people who had complete cytogenetic remission at the time of the trial—if you look at people who are at complete cytogenetic remission at six months, like you are, this is probably less than 5 percent, so—"

"Over four years?"

"Yeah," the doctor replied. "Now, if you look at the curves, truth be known, there's a steady decline. It's about a risk of losing progression overall in the study of somewhere between 2 and 4 percent per year."

"Say that part again," the patient interjects, "because I didn't quite follow you."

The patient is understandably confused. In less than two minutes time she has been deluged with numbers—80 percent, 15 percent, forty-eight months, four years. Whose head wouldn't be spinning? Later in this conversation, during an appointment that lasted more than an hour, the patient would learn that if she goes into complete remission (one of those numbers from above, I think), she would still face a 5 percent risk of cancer progression over the next four years, and a 4 percent risk (time frame unspecified by the physician) of expressing new chromosomal changes. If she has a recurrence, she can get a bone marrow transplant (which led to a five- or ten-minute conversation laying out the odds of surviving such a treatment, plus the odds of experiencing graft-versus-host disease: "There's about a 40 to 50 percent chance you'd need some therapy for that. And then if you are an unrelated donor and a match, it goes up to about 70 percent"), with the subsequent risk of chronic relapse of 5 to 8 percent depending on . . . well, does it really matter anymore?

We physicians are a highly numerate group of people. To us, numbers are second nature. In many doctor–patient encounters, in fact, physicians unwittingly flip back and forth between percentages (3 percent) and frequencies (8 out of 100). After all, isn't 3 percent the same thing as 3 out of 100? But for many patients, this back and forth is incredibly confusing. Look what this back and forth did to Yogi Berra, who, when asked by reporters to explain the intricacies of baseball, said that "90 percent of the game is half mental."

Many laypeople, in fact, have difficulty with some of the most basic properties of mathematics. For instance, Steven Woloshin and Lisa Schwartz, physicians at Dartmouth who study risk communication, asked laypeople questions like "If you flipped a fair coin a thousand times, how many times would it land on heads?" They discovered that almost a third of people don't answer correctly. In short, there are lots of reasons to be concerned that newly empowered patients will make bad decisions—decisions that are not in their best interests, decisions that they would take back if they could—because they are confused about the math.

But our concerns about patients' decisions should not end with innumeracy, because the challenges people face in making wise choices, in factoring numerical risks into their decisions, go well beyond mere confusion about percentages and frequencies. Take the colon cancer scenario I described earlier, in which the majority of people choose a treatment that increases their chance of dying just so they can avoid treatment complications that are preferable to death. We assessed numeracy among people making this strange choice and discovered that people who were good at math were just as likely to make this choice as people who weren't so good. What's more, we circulated this decision to physicians across the United States and discovered almost half of them chose the uncomplicated surgery too.

Trust me. Every physician who made that choice had a robust comprehension of what 4 percent means. Every single one of them understood the trade-off between death and colostomy. And I cannot believe that any of them truly believed they would rather be dead than live with diarrhea or a temporary wound infection. That means their choices were not about comprehension. Instead, their choices reveal that even when people understand the numbers, the way those numbers make people feel can still influence their decisions.

It's because of these feelings that I relayed the hematologist's conversation. That hematologist made some of the mistakes we saw in chapter 3: enough jargon to drown a battleship. But in addition, that hematologist overlooked the way numbers make people feel.

Consider a study led by Ellen Peters, a psychologist at the Ohio State University. Peters gave research volunteers a chance to win money by selecting a jelly bean at random from one of two bowls. The catch? They would only win if they got lucky and pulled out a red jelly bean. To help people decide which bowl to choose from, Peters put a label on one of the bowls indicating that it contained 9 percent (9 out of 100) red jelly beans and on the other bowl indicating that it contained 10 percent (1 out of 10) red jelly beans. The choice here is straightforward, because 10 percent is bigger than 9 percent. But many people feel conflicted by this choice, because there's only one red bean in the 10 percent bowl, and 9 of them in the 9 percent bowl. People *know* that they ought to choose from the 10 percent bowl, but many of them still *feel* tempted to choose from the 9 percent bowl, because 9 out of 100 seems bigger than 1 out of 10.

Not surprisingly, the worse people are at math, the more likely they are to choose from the 9 percent bowl. But their choice is not merely a matter of comprehension. It's also about emotion. People who struggle at math, even when they know the right answer, feel less confident about the answer. Their attraction to the bigger bowl, the one with more red jelly beans in it, is harder to resist. Throw enough numbers at people and many will experience negative emotions, emotions that often interfere with their ability to make good choices.

A PILL TO PREVENT BREAST CANCER

Her mom had developed breast cancer at age seventy-two, and now Juliette Evans contemplated her own risk of that disease. Sitting in front of her computer, she had answered a series of questions about her medical history: how old she was when she had her first baby, how old she was when she started menstruating. The questions were ones my colleagues and I had posed so that we could calculate her chance of developing breast cancer over the next five years. From her answers, we estimated that she faced a 3 percent chance of being diagnosed with breast cancer over that time period.

Why on earth would we want to calculate this risk? Because we wanted to help women like Evans decide whether to take a pill that would reduce their chance of developing breast cancer. Evans had used her computer to access a decision aid my colleagues and I had developed to introduce women to the risks and benefits of two medicines, raloxifene and tamoxifen, which had been proven to reduce the occurrence of breast cancer in women who, while they hadn't yet experienced a cancer diagnosis, nevertheless faced a substantial risk of breast cancer over the next five years. (I will tell you more about decision aids in part III, but for now think of them as very robust, well-designed educational brochures.)

I realize that 3 percent might not strike readers as a very "substantial" risk. But most of you reading this book, especially if you are as young as Evans was when she read our decision aid, don't face a 3 percent risk of any serious illness over the next five years. Only fifty-six years old at the time, Evans was not in any mood to face a potentially life-threatening disease. But what could she do about that 3 percent risk?

She could continue to receive annual mammograms. But mammograms don't prevent cancer. They identify cancers at an early stage, presumably in time so that some of those cancers will be cured before becoming life threatening. She could continue performing breast self-exams. But those have no proven benefit, even in improving the cure rate of cancers. Exercise and diet, too, don't really do much to prevent breast cancer. So if Evans wanted to reduce her risk, she either needed to choose a drastic intervention, like having her breasts prophylactically removed, or she needed to take one of these pills.

What are the benefits of raloxifene and tamoxifen? With these medicines, Evans's risk of developing breast cancer over the next five years would be cut in half. To put that in perspective, tamoxifen and raloxifene were as good at preventing breast cancer as most cholesterol pills are at preventing heart attacks. But of course there was a catch. The pills carried a risk of unpleasant side effects. Odds were close to even that Evans would at least temporarily experience symptoms that reminded her of menopause—hot flashes and mood swings, a desire to maim her husband, things like that. She'd face a less than 1 in 100 chance of experiencing serious blood clots, potentially leading to a heart attack or stroke. Even less likely, but surely something to ponder, was a 2 in 1,000 chance that she would develop endometrial cancer. Her doctor would monitor her for all of these potential side effects. In the case of endometrial cancer, there was almost no chance the cancer would slip out of their control before they could cure it. But still, not a pleasant complication to ponder.

Our decision aid laid out all of this information for Evans in clear, precise language. No worries about medical terminology being lost in translation; the decision aid had been scrubbed clean by a literacy expert. Short sentences, plenty of white space, every term defined in seventh-grade language. No rush to judgment either. We repeatedly informed women perusing our decision aid that they could read and reread the materials at their leisure, even share the information with loved ones and talk things over with their doctors.

But had our decision aid improved her decision making? Or had we been too busy informing her about the risks and benefits of these medicines to pay attention to how those risks and benefits would make her feel?

COMPARED TO WHOM?

Nearly a dozen women sat around the conference room table with drafts of our decision aid printed out for their perusal. A facilitator was seated among them to solicit their feedback.

"Where do these risk numbers come from?" a woman asked.

The facilitator explained that the numbers were individualized for each person, based on their medical and family history. That means some women looking at the decision aid would learn that their five-year risk is 3 percent while others might learn it's 2, 4, or 5 percent.

"That's all fine," the woman responded, "but what good is that information without knowledge of the average woman's risk?" Others chimed in, echoing her question. "Is 3 percent high or low?" they wanted to know. "Is it above average or below?"

The facilitator nodded, unable to answer their questions. Her job was to see how women responded to the decision aid and report her observations back to my colleagues and me.

A near-universal desire had surfaced in this focus group. These women wouldn't be satisfied merely with individualized information about the risk of breast cancer, or even with the subsequent information about how tamoxifen and raloxifene reduced that risk; in addition, they wanted information about how their risk of breast cancer compared to that of the average woman.

Seems like a reasonable enough request, one we could accommodate with a minor modification of our decision aid. Yet I was hesitant to make this modification. I wasn't sure this comparative-risk information was relevant to their decisions. If a woman faced a 3 percent risk of breast cancer in the next five years, she needed to decide whether cutting that risk in half was a large enough benefit to justify the risks and burdens of these medications. If her risk of breast cancer were 3 percent over the next five years, would it matter if the average woman's risk were 4 percent? Or 24 percent, for that matter? Nothing about the average woman's risk would change anything about the risks and benefits she needed to consider in order to make this decision.

As the relevance of comparative-risk information bounced around my brain, I found myself unwilling to add this information to our decision aid. At least not before I had a chance to run an experiment. Unwilling for ethical reasons to experiment on women who were actively contemplating this decision, I recruited what we in the research world call a "convenience sample" of women and asked each of them to imagine, purely hypothetically, that they faced a 6 percent risk of breast cancer over the next five years. Additionally, I asked some of them to imagine that the average woman faced only a 3 percent risk over that same time period. This group of women, in other words, thought of the 6 percent risk as being double that of the average woman. And I asked another group of women to imagine that the average woman faced a 12 percent risk. In their minds, then, these women perceived the 6 percent risk as half the normal risk. Then I asked all of these women to make a hypothetical choice: Would they take a pill that would cut their 6 percent risk of breast cancer in half, to 3 percent, but would also cause them to experience those side effects I described above—unpleasant things like menopausal symptoms?

As I feared, women's interest in the pill depended on whether they believed their risk was above or below average. Those women who were randomized to the above-average risk group were significantly more interested in taking tamoxifen and believed, in fact, that tamoxifen was more effective than did the women who were made to believe that their risk was below average. The same number—6 percent—felt significantly more worrisome when it represented an above-average risk, the kind of risk women felt they should take action against. When that 6 percent figure represented a below-average risk, however, it prompted much less sense of urgency, the kind of risk that compels neither action nor anxiety.

Comparative-risk information changes the way people think and feel about risk. And its influence reveals a vital truth about risk statistics, that the same number can feel very different to different people due to subtle differences in the emotional context of that risk information.

This phenomenon explains how a group of well-intentioned medical educators unwittingly caused a group of previously anxious women to become strangely unconcerned about breast cancer. These educators set out to help women understand the risks and benefits of mammograms, believing like most proponents of the new paradigm that such understanding would lead to better decision making. They began by assessing women's knowledge, asking them, for example, what they believed their lifetime chances were of being diagnosed with breast cancer. The educators' assessment uncovered widespread confusion. The average woman faces a 13 percent risk of being diagnosed with breast cancer in her lifetime, but this group of women mistakenly believed that their risks were much, much higher—30 percent, 40 percent, even 50 percent.

Enter educators stage left, armed with facts and plain-language pamphlets. The educators explained to each woman what her actual risk was of developing breast cancer and what parts of her medical and family history contributed to this risk. And their educational efforts succeeded, with women now spouting off their true risk like it was a long-known fact. But the education also produced an unforeseen side effect. It caused women to lose interest in mammograms!

Think about what happened here. Imagine that you believed, prior to receiving the educational intervention, that you faced a 40 percent chance of developing breast cancer in your lifetime. Wouldn't a 13 percent risk feel pretty small?

It is tempting to state that the new paradigm failed these women, that it was misguided to educate them about their health risks. It is also tempting to argue that the new paradigm served these women well, helping them realize that their risk of breast cancer was too low to justify a painful and inconvenient mammogram. But I know better than to draw either of these conclusions from this fiasco. I know better because I conducted an experiment. I began the experiment by asking one group of women to estimate their lifetime risk of developing breast cancer. The women guessed, on average, that their risk was around 40 percent. And just like those women in the education study, the women in my study were quite relieved to learn of the 13 percent figure, breathing a sigh of relief and telling me that the risk felt low.

But my study didn't end there, because at the same time that I asked this group of women to guess their risk of breast cancer, I selected another group of women at random from the same pool and gave them the 13 percent figure up front, without first asking them to guess their risk. This group felt quite differently about the 13 percent figure, finding it anxiety provoking, nothing to be relieved about at all. By the end of my experiment, these two groups had identical knowledge of their breast cancer risks, understanding that the average risk was 13 percent. But their reaction to this risk information was dramatically different, simply because one group had been asked to guess the number before learning it.

When patients face difficult medical choices, they need to understand their alternatives. But their ultimate decisions depend on more than their understanding of such facts; they're also influenced by subtle contextual cues that change how the risks and benefits of these alternatives feel. A 6 percent risk will feel different from a 6 in 100 risk, which will feel different from a 60 in 1,000 risk, all of which will feel different when contrasted with an average person's risk or the average person's average guess of the average risk, or . . . well, you get the picture.

The new paradigm of patient self-determination and autonomy has not taken full account of the psychology of medical decision making. According to the new paradigm, patients have a moral right to comprehensible information about their medical alternatives. But which way of presenting such information is morally appropriate? Is it okay to tell someone her risk is 6,000 out of 100,000? Or is that figure too alarming? Is any number neutral?

CLARITY OF VISION

The kinds of decisions people face in medical contexts are in so many ways different from the decisions they confront in other aspects of their lives. When I make my biannual trip to the mall to buy clothes, I can quickly peruse the shelves of shirts and find colors, fabrics, and prices that suit my preferences. Occasionally, I purchase a shirt that falls apart on the fourth wearing, not altogether surprising given my proclivity for deeply discounted apparel. Rarely a shirt will shrink more than expected and my oldest son will gain another dad-me-down for his wardrobe. But I pretty much know what I like, shirt-wise, after all these years, and the stakes of bad decisions are so low that it doesn't really matter if I occasionally make a bad choice.

My shirt-shopping choices are as different from medical choices as choices can be—low stakes, devoid of emotion (other than my general displeasure at spending time at malls), no difficult numbers to process, repeated exposure to the same basic choice many times in my life, and temporary consequences with plenty of opportunity to correct bad decisions. Nothing in common with, say, a decision about whether to undergo a below-the-knee amputation rather than spend more time with a painful foot ulcer that refuses to bow to antibiotics. Nothing in common with the choice between surgery and radiation, for someone with a newly diagnosed cancer.

Yet in other ways medical decisions aren't so different from other decisions. For example, I am typically at the mercy of auto mechanics when they tell me what is wrong with my '99 Accord. Like a patient interacting with a physician, I am much less knowledgeable about the situation at hand than the expert advising me. Medical decisions are a bit like mortgage shopping too, with a confusing array of statistics that lie outside many people's grasp: a 4 percent adjustable rate that has a 50 percent chance of rising two or more points over the next three years, at which time my payments could grow from . . . sigh.

Faced with these kinds of decisions—ones that involve complex information and confusing trade-offs—people often try to focus on the information most important for making their choice. But often, identifying that information is a challenge. Imagine that you are searching the Internet for information on ophthalmologists, in hopes of receiving laser surgery to correct your nearsightedness. You come across two promising candidates.

The first ophthalmologist is Dr. Bettereyes. Educated at Harvard Medical School, he uses a next-generation excimer laser, which he purchased last year. Dr. Bettereyes reports on his website that he has performed this type of eye surgery over 80 times with excellent results.

The second doctor you find is Dr. Seebetter, who was educated at the University of Iowa and who uses the same kind of excimer laser as Bettereyes. He reports on his website that he has performed this procedure over 300 times with excellent results.

Which doctor would you choose? When my colleague Brian Zikmund-Fisher and I presented this hypothetical choice to people, almost everyone gave higher ratings to the Iowa-trained doctor, impressed by his experience with this new technology. (In fact, there is only one university where I have presented this study that a majority of the audience gave the other doctor higher ratings. Care to guess which one?) But when we gave a separate group of people information about only one of these two doctors, some getting information about the Harvard doctor and others getting information about the Iowa doctor, the Harvard doctor received higher average ratings than the Iowa doctor.

In isolation, the Harvard doctor received higher ratings because his experience—80 procedures—was hard to evaluate. Is 80 a lot or a little? Without comparison information about other doctors, it's hard for people to judge. We know that the doctor isn't a total newbie at the procedure, but we don't know if 80 signifies a substantial amount of experience. Harvard, on the other hand, is easy for people to evaluate—it is obviously a prestigious school. Only after people have access to information about the Iowa physician does the experience level of the Harvard doctor became easier to evaluate and, in this case, less impressive.

When patients find themselves faced with important medical decisions, they often lack the kind of contextual information they need to evaluate their alternatives. A 3 percent risk of cancer over the next five years is very difficult information for people to contextualize. How many times in our lives have any of us pondered our risk of something bad happening to us over that particular time frame? We shouldn't be surprised to discover that, when patients are given such information by medical practitioners enthused about the new paradigm of patient empowerment, most will eagerly seek out ways to place that information into context. The downside of such eagerness is that whatever contextual information happens to be available often ends up having a huge influence on their thinking, sometimes for the better (giving them enough context to judge a doctor's amount of experience, for instance) but other times for the worse (informing them about other people's risks, even when such information has no bearing on their own).

Patient empowerment can come at a price, overwhelming patients with alternatives, confusing them with numerical data that they lack appropriate context to evaluate. As we've seen, numbers create feelings, and the context in which people receive risk information can cause the same, say, 6 percent risk to feel small or large. To make matters worse, the emotion created by a decision can also change how a risk feels.

SHOCKING FEELINGS

The electrode clamped to your forearm has just delivered a jolt to your system, a surge of electricity that is perfectly safe yet completely unpleasant. How unpleasant? Well you wouldn't pay fifty dollars to avoid another jolt, but you'd spend as much as twenty dollars.

Now let's play a probability game. To show how it works, let's put aside electrical shocks for a moment and concentrate instead on money. Suppose I've just given you twenty dollars, and I'm about to spin a wheel that gives me a 99 percent chance of taking all of that money back from you. How much will you pay to stop me from spinning the wheel? If you are like most people, you will spend as much as seventeen or eighteen dollars to keep from losing all of your newfound cash. Suppose, instead, the wheel gives me only a 1 percent chance to take back the twenty dollars. In this case, most people will part with no more than one dollar to guarantee the remainder of their money.

What have we learned from the game? For starters, if we mapped out people's payments across the entire range of odds—from a 1 percent chance of losing to a 99 percent chance—we would see that their payments make relatively big jumps when the odds shift from zero percent to 1 percent, and from 99 percent to 100 percent. If I have no chance of losing, if the wheel is rigged in my favor, I won't pay a cent to keep you from spinning the wheel. But a 1 percent chance of losing all twenty dollars? Most people will pay more than 1 percent of their money to avoid the gamble. In technical terms, decision experts would conclude that the relationship between probability and money in this game isn't completely linear.

I bring up these monetary gambles not to highlight differences between the way people feel toward money and electric shocks. When it comes to electric shocks, people will pay that same twenty dollars to avoid a 100 percent chance of being shocked, but they will also pay a whopping seven dollars to avoid a 1 percent chance. When people contemplate emotional events like a 1 percent chance of being shocked, that 1 percent risk exerts a large influence on their behavior. Consider the colon cancer scenario described earlier in this chapter; the strong emotions elicited by contemplation of colostomies and infected wounds caused people to opt for the uncomplicated surgery, the thought of the colostomy operating like an electric shock, causing people to treat low probabilities like they are much larger probabilities—so unpleasant to contemplate that *any* chance of a colostomy is too big of a chance to take.

In fact, my colleagues and I decided to test whether colostomies are like electrical shocks (in how they distort the way low-probability events feel to people) by conducting a simple experiment. We gave one group of people a direct (and extremely hypothetical!) choice between certain death and a colostomy. In this case, most people said they would opt for the colostomy. We gave the second group of people a different choice (again, as with everything I refer to as an experiment, the two groups are random subsets of the same population): between a 4 percent risk of death and a 4 percent risk of colostomy. In this uncertain situation, a significant number of people told us they would choose death over colostomy. Colostomies did create electric shock–like reactions in people, with a colostomy looming relatively large over their decision, even when described as a rare event. Icky things, no matter how rare, are powerful motivators.

These thought experiments would be nothing more than academic exercises but for the fact that they reveal psychological forces that I have witnessed scores of times in my medical practice, when emotionally evocative treatment outcomes have caused my patients to act in ways that even they know are not in their best interests. Health-care decision making is rife, after all, with evocative images—needles and syringes, unsettling sights and odious odors. I cannot tell you how many of my patients have refused insulin therapy for their diabetes because such treatment would involve daily injections. Nor can I count the number of patients I have counseled who decline to take beneficial medications due to fear of rare but emotionally charged complications. The feel of risk almost always wins out over cold, hard statistics.

BODY OF EVIDENCE

Emotion also influences medical decisions in another surprising way, which I will illustrate by describing a clever study.

The study begins like a jewelry store heist, with a laser beam stretched across the room, except that moving across the path of this beam does not set off alarms or trigger a sudden locking of impenetrable doors. Researchers have set up these laser beams to create an excuse for directing people to move their bodies in ways that reveal the surprising power of emotional gestures to shape people's thinking. The experimenters told the research participants that they were studying the effect of muscle movement on reading. Under this guise, they instructed participants to wave their arms up and down through the path of the laser beam upon their command.

"Extend digit A," the researchers would command, and participants would raise their thumb like a thumbs-up sign and lift their arm up and down through the beam. "Now extend digit B," and up rose participants' index fingers. "Digit C," and now participants' middle fingers would be extended, their arms moving up and down as if they were flipping off the world.

The flipping-off part was actually the point of the researchers' strange instructions. They had tricked participants into making emotionally evocative gestures, to see how such bodily movements would influence thinking. The participants had been reading a description of an ambiguously aggressive man named Donald, a man described as having refused to pay his rent because the landlord had failed to make promised repairs on his apartment.

Those people who read about Donald while raising digit C, their middle finger, thought much worse of him than those who read about him while raising digit A, their thumb. Unbeknownst to the participants, when they were sticking up their middle finger, for reasons that had nothing to do with their emotions, it nevertheless created an emotion that then influenced the way they judged the actions of this hypothetical character.

The way people feel inevitably shapes their judgments and decisions. Ask people to hold a pen between their eyes while making a judgment, a feat that can only be accomplished by furrowing their brows, and they make more negative judgments. The brow furrowing influences their attitudes, even though the furrowing is unrelated to their evaluation. Arrange for a random set of people to find a dime before answering a survey, and they will indicate on the survey that they have much higher life satisfaction. Conduct the same survey in an uncomfortably warm room, and their overall life satisfaction will plunge, the uncomfortable feeling contaminating their judgments.

If you feel bad when making a risky decision, or if something about the job of making the decision makes you feel bad, then that bad feeling will spill over onto the way you judge the risks at hand. This spillover of feeling onto judgment is a huge challenge for anyone trying to make good medical decisions. For instance, when a patient reads a drug information label printed in an uncomfortably small font, she will experience stress. This distress will cause her to judge the medication as being more risky. If the same medication is given an easy-to-pronounce name, patients will judge it as less harmful than if its name is harder to pronounce. The mere effort of figuring out the name of the drug causes people to look for reasons to dislike it. No wonder so many patients prefer expensive trade drugs over hard-to-pronounce generics.

THE PLACE OF EMOTIONS IN MAKING WISE CHOICES

Oscar Wilde once quipped, "The advantage of emotions is that they lead us astray." Indeed, what fun would life be if we didn't at least occasionally get carried away by our emotions—date that girl who's going to break our heart, make a fool of ourselves at an outrageous party? Wilde's take on emotions, though, is a caricature of emotion, with logic inevitably pointing us in the right direction if we can only keep our emotions in check. My discussion of feelings in this chapter may reinforce the stereotype of emotions as a bad influence, but that is not at all my point. Emotions don't inevitably lead people astray. In fact, they frequently play an important role in helping people make good decisions.

For example, people whose emotional functioning has been damaged by injury or illness often make terrible decisions, even when their ability to reason is intact. Antonio Damasio famously made this point in his influential book *Descartes' Error*. Damasio has conducted a slew of creative studies on patients with damage to their frontal lobes, people whose higher level cognition is intact, who can calculate the odds of just about anything and tell you with decision-analytic precision the choice that best serves their interests, but who frequently fail to make logical choices. They know the right choice to make, but because they don't simultaneously *feel* it's the right choice, they don't follow through on their own reasoning. Emotions, after all, evolved for a reason. Often when things don't feel right, it's because they aren't right.

I bring up Damasio's research to highlight an important point. Emotions are neither good nor bad for decision making; they are both good and bad. Sometimes they lead us astray and other times they point us in the right direction. My goal in writing about emotions and decision making is to raise a question about patient self-determination. Emotions play a huge role in the decisions we all make; often in ways so subtle we are unaware of their influence.

This lack of awareness is my real concern, because the new paradigm of patient-based decision making rose up from a world almost devoid of emotion. Bioethicists and lawyers wrote eloquently about the centrality of individual rights, of patient autonomy in medical decision making, laying out criteria for informed choice. Patients have a right to comprehensible information so that they can integrate such information with their values in order to make choices that promote their individual versions of the good life. In 1990, for example, the U.S. government passed what it called the Patient Self-Determination Act, a law requiring hospitals and other health-care organizations to provide patients with information about advanced health-care directives, so patients can decide up front what they want done if they become too sick to make their own medical decisions. The government also pushed for health-care institutions to create ethics review boards, IRBs, which now spend much of their time obsessing over the specific language in consent forms, to ensure that patients have the right information available when they make their decisions. Regulators at the FDA have pushed hard to require pharmaceutical companies to include thorough side-effect information on drug safety labels. The new paradigm is built on a foundation of rational choice, an edifice whose stability depends on the idea that information and freedom lead to optimal decision making.

But in the midst of all these important issues of morality and law, there is rarely a word about emotion. Proponents of the new paradigm have been so focused on giving patients access to information that they've not paid enough attention to how this information makes patients feel.

TAKING MEASURE

In the previous four chapters, I have taken measure of how doctors and patients are stumbling their way through the new paradigm of shared decision making. Some physicians, intent on informing patients about their medical alternatives, end up overwhelming them with jargon, all the while oblivious to their emotional desires and needs. Many patients are oblivious too. They believe they've understood their doctor's words, even when they haven't. They think they know what it will feel like to experience a colostomy, even when they don't. And they are completely unaware of subtle psychological phenomena that dramatically alter the way they feel about unlikely events.

All these issues—these miscommunications, misperceptions, and misimaginings—come into play in even relatively mundane medical encounters: hypertensive patients mistakenly believing that they can feel when their blood pressure is elevated, diabetes patients convinced that they will never get used to injecting themselves with daily insulin, primary care doctors confident that they have conveyed the importance of colon cancer screening to patients who will find excuses not to schedule their colonoscopy exams.

Soon, I will start laying out steps doctors and patients can take to improve these matters, to work together to make better decisions. But we don't yet have the full measure of our challenge, and without a more complete understanding of just how poorly the new paradigm is working, we won't know what it will take to rectify the situation. To get a more complete measure of where we stand, we need to explore what happens when the stakes are highest, when the decisions doctors and patients make are truly matters of life and death.

SEVEN

Back and Forth over Life and Death

He'd lost so much weight the baby fat had long ago left his face. Even his muscles had wasted away; his face was now dominated by a pair of prominent cheekbones protruding beneath sunken skin. The lung cancer had already spread to Doug Stevens's brain and was continuing to grow, despite aggressive chemotherapy. And now he was back in the hospital with a life-threatening pneumonia, an infection caused by the tumor masses still residing in his already damaged lungs.

I had read in Stevens's medical chart about his battle with cancer and about the tepid way his body had responded to chemotherapy. I had reviewed his X-rays and CT scans, six months of tumor progression documented in time-lapse photography, like one of those nature shows where a flower sprouts and blooms in front of your eyes, weeks of growth fast-forwarded in the space of a few seconds. I'd examined his frail physique and listened to what was left of his lungs. It was clear to me that he was near the end of his life. Now I wanted to find out what was clear to him.

"What have your doctors been telling you about your illness?" I asked.

"They said they couldn't cure me, but they could treat me."

"What do you think that means?"

"I don't know," he replied. "I guess it means I still have hope."

"What kind of hope?"

"Maybe they can stop the cancer. Do you think?"

Treat but not cure. I found myself pondering that idea in the context of Stevens's sad situation. I had used those words hundreds of times in my career, one of my go-to phrases to let patients with chronic diseases know that they were in it for the long haul, that their illness wasn't going away, and that they needed to reconcile themselves to lifelong therapy. I had communicated this idea to people with adult-onset diabetes, most of who would remain diabetic for the rest of their lives. I had uttered it to people with high blood pressure, people who might otherwise believe that their hypertension would behave like a winter bronchitis—ten days of pills and life would return to normal.

But what does it mean to convey this idea to a man with terminal cancer?

In this man's case, the idea of "treat but not cure" was true in a literal sense. We could irradiate his lungs and possibly shrink whatever part of the tumor was contributing to his pneumonia. We could switch to a new chemotherapy, in hopes of slowing his cancer down for a few weeks. But Stevens's cancer was incurable from the get-go, from the day six months earlier when he had developed blurry vision and his doctor had discovered a pair of metastases in his brain. All of his doctors had known back then that no treatment would stop the tumors from growing and spreading. It would be a miracle if he survived even a year.

And now he lay in a hospital bed, tossing a phrase around in his mind—"we can treat your cancer"—and holding out hope that he could live to retirement age with well-contained tumors no longer threatening his life.

END-OF-LIFE DECISION MAKING:
A WINDOW TO THE REVOLUTION

Revolutions rarely begin in a specific place, at one moment in time. But they often begin quickly and focally enough to have starting places. The American Revolution largely began in the Northern colonies, with the Continental Congress in Philadelphia, the Tea Party in Boston, and the shots fired at Lexington and Concord. The patient-empowerment revolution also began relatively focally, at the bedsides of dying patients. Lawyers didn't start the revolution by taking doctors to court for prescribing blood pressure medicines without adequate consent. Nor did bioethicists establish their stake in the debate by setting up commissions to determine how to involve patients in decisions about treating upper-respiratory infections. Instead, the revolution centered on high-stakes situations, on clashes between patients (and their families) and their clinicians about when to pull the plug, about whether to hasten the end, and about what it means for end-of-life care to be "futile."

The end of life is when the revolution began, with Karen Ann Quinlan's case, followed by a whole bevy of end-of-life judicial rulings, cases that grabbed the attention of health lawyers, bioethicists, and clinicians focused on "pull the plug" dramas. As important as it is for patients to be involved in choosing whether to take, say, cholesterol pills, such decisions hardly compare to battles over whether families should be able to remove feeding tubes from their loved ones or whether burn victims, early in the course of their painful treatments, should be able to stop treatment and die, despite high odds of achieving a meaningful recovery.

When I trained in clinical ethics in the early 1990s, the lion's share of my course work focused on end-of-life decision making. Most of the ethics consults I performed at that time centered on desperately ill patients at odds with their oncologists or their ICU physicians about

aggressive treatments. No surprise, really, that many of my physician colleagues who have remained active as bioethicists now practice palliative-care medicine, a specialty devoted to easing suffering
among people who are near the end of their lives.

Leaders of the revolution have focused much of their energy on
improving end-of-life care. They successfully lobbied for federal legislation, the Patient Self-Determination Act, which requires hospitals
to ask patients whether they have living wills. They have conducted
multimillion-dollar studies testing out methods to reduce unnecessary use of CPR at the end of life. They have worked to promote the
hospice movement and the field of palliative care, to balance out the
aggressive treatment-focused specialties otherwise dominating medical care.

Ironic, then, that much of what I've explored so far—the overcom-
munication and undercommunication, the impenetrable jargon, the
emotions interfering with clear thinking, the whole struggle between
persuasion and neutrality—all become so much more difficult in the
setting of end-of-life care. Dire medical situations create a set of needs
and desires among both patients and physicians that conspire against
good decision making, causing patients to seek out hope where none
exists, to hear "hope" when little has been communicated. All of this
hopefulness even changes the way doctors think and talk about these
same situations.

If we want to understand the state of the revolution and how we
might best help our loved ones going through it, we need to dig
deeper into the world of end-of-life decision making. If we wish to
grasp the barriers that stand in the way of shared decision making, we
need to return to the place where the revolution began: the bedside of
patients who feel as if they have nothing to lose.

HANGING CREPE OR PLANNING FOR A PARTY?

She's dead. That was my first thought upon seeing her chest X-ray. Kate Bauer's right lung was almost entirely whited out (a normal lung, being filled mostly with air, looks dark on an X-ray), the tissue overrun by what looked like a combination of tumor and infection. A heavy smoker for thirty years, with a voice resembling the older version of Lucille Ball, she had lost weight over the previous three months and had come to me feeling "just a bit run down."

I didn't believe, of course, that she was already literally dead. I didn't even think her demise was imminent. Instead, a more drawn out worst-case scenario leapt out at me from her X-ray. It was as if, in an instant, I could see her future. A biopsy, probably through a bronchoscope, would confirm the specific identity of the tumor invading her emphysematous lungs, and maybe even identify which antibiotic would overcome the related pneumonia. We would clear up the infection, maybe give her some treatment or chemotherapy, but given the overall state of her aggressively abused body, she would be lucky to live six months.

A colleague walked past the X-ray image. "Oh, she's screwed," he said.

I turned away from the image and walked toward the exam room, pondering what to tell Ms. Bauer about her X-ray. How do I tell her she's screwed? By saying no such thing, of course. That would not only be cruel but also premature. The mass visible on her chest X-ray was highly suspicious of a malignancy, almost "pathognomonic"—consistent with almost nothing else. But "almost" was the key concept shaping my words that day. I knew it was cancer, a gut-feeling kind of knowledge that wouldn't cut the mustard in a freshman philosophy seminar. I knew, but I didn't really know. True knowledge would require more evidence—tissue is the issue, as we internists like to say. And there was a remote chance her illness was something unusual.

Anything, I reminded myself halfheartedly, can present as tuberculosis; maybe she has a curable infection.

So I reentered the exam room and immediately launched into an optimistic description of the likely infection compromising her current health. I explained that much of her right lung was consumed by the infection and that, if (when! I probably said "when") we got the infection under control, she would feel significantly better. Then, her spirits now rising a little more than I'd hoped, I broke the bad news:

"Now, the real question is why you have this infection. The X-ray shows a shadow, a growth you could say." You could say? "And this growth may be what caused your lung to get infected."

How's that for clarity? Yet she understood what I was saying. "Cancer, then?" she asked resolutely. "I have cancer?"

"We don't know that," I quickly interjected. "This could be any number of things." (Things? Amazingly eloquent, aren't I?) "This could be some other thing altogether, something we can take care of so you can get back on your feet."

"Oh, Dr. Ubel, you don't have to worry. I've smoked my whole life. This is how it was bound to end."

"Nothing is ending here," I countered. "We just have to treat this infection and then we'll figure out what other problems we need to take care of." She gave me a knowing look, leaving me to feel like a child who had just lied about practicing piano.

Had I done anything wrong? I hadn't lied to her. I'd simply begun a process of managing her expectations, of delivering kind-of-bad but not oh-God-it's-over news, so she wouldn't be overwhelmed. I was being cautious, not deceptive, making sure not to jump the gun. Nevertheless, I felt dishonest. Looking at her X-ray out in the workroom, I had as much as declared her dead. Now I found myself looking for ways to keep her from coming to the same conclusion. Why did I feel so determined to put a positive spin on her situation?

LOOKING FOR HOPE IN ALL THE WRONG PLACES

Nixon never went so far as to officially declare it a war. But due to all the cash he threw at the National Cancer Institute in the early 1970s, he is credited for being the commander in chief at the beginning of the war on cancer. Forty years later, the war continues with some notable victories under our belts. Most childhood cancers, for example, are curable now. Some adult cancers too, like testicular cancer. Even when that disease is widely metastasized, as it was in Lance Armstrong's case, the majority of people can be cured. There has also been tremendous progress preventing cancer, most notably through successful antitobacco campaigns.

But most cancers remain as deadly now as they were forty years ago. When cancers metastasize in places like the lungs, the liver, or the pancreas, when they spread beyond the boundaries of their home organs, they are virtually unstoppable. Surgery, chemotherapy, and radiation may slow down such tumors for a while, but these metastasized tumors usually bounce back and win. In the meantime, these desperate treatments are often quite toxic. They attack cancer by targeting cellular reproduction. Cancers spread because cancer cells reproduce more rapidly than normal cells. Disturb such reproduction and the cancers won't spread as rapidly. However, cancer cells are not alone in reproducing. Hair cells like to replicate frequently; that's why so many chemotherapies make people bald. Gastrointestinal cells typically replicate frequently too, which explains why so many people undergoing chemotherapy suffer from nausea and diarrhea.

So the decision to treat an incurable cancer is fraught with difficult trade-offs. The extra months of life gained through treatment may come at the cost of months of misery. Unrealistic hope in the face of a death sentence isn't some benevolent balm, soothing people at a time of need. The wrong kind of optimism can cause patients to put themselves through treatments that will only increase their misery.

Yet too often I have found myself doing everything in my power to help patients find hope in hopeless situations. Each year, I spend a month caring for hospitalized patients in the VA system, and in that brief time I inevitably immerse myself in the ends of a couple dozen lives. So many of the patients on the general medical wards have dismally predictable futures, with end-stage illnesses eating away at their fading bodies.

On the first day of my month in the hospital, my team of residents, interns, and students typically walks the corridors with me, telling me each patient's story in the hallway before we step inside the room to meet each one. The residents and interns—who, because I cover the hospital in January, have spent the better part of six months working in the hospital, nary a week going by without one of their patients dying—often have a look of worn-out resignation; the death and dying is taking its toll. Medical students, by contrast, many of whom are in their first month on an internal medicine team, don't look resigned so much as shocked, and overwhelmed by gloom and doom.

Why am I telling you about doctors' feelings and the challenges of hospital work when it's the patients who face the real challenges? Because part of the context of end-of-life decision making results from doctors' emotions. During my inpatient months, I would quickly find myself feeling down about the awful illnesses my patients were suffering from, and my response would be to find some way, almost any way, to feel better. I'd discover myself lingering a bit longer at the bedsides of healthier, happier patients. I'd find myself marveling at the great turnaround made by the person with congestive heart failure in room 503. And I'd notice myself putting off the difficult conversations that I knew needed to take place in rooms 506 and 511, rooms with patients whose cancers were advancing rapidly despite aggressive treatment.

Worse yet, when I did get around to talking to such patients, I'd find myself dismissing their pessimistic prognostications—the fears they'd express about dying, for example—with absurd and inaccurate clichés: "You're not dying anytime soon. We're going to make you better!"

There's a joke we primary care docs like to tell each other. "Why do coffins have nails?" we ask. The answer is "to keep out the oncologists." From our perch in the outpatient clinics, we primary care doctors have seen too many of our patients hospitalized by oncologists for "salvage chemotherapy," a toxic therapy that rips out patients' insides at the same time that it rips them away from family and friends. (Salvage chemotherapy is treatment that is given after a tumor recurs despite earlier treatment.) We wise generalists scoff at our subspecialty colleagues for losing sight of patients' quality of life.

Within hours of beginning my monthly hospital duties, that coffin joke would stop being quite so funny, for I would find myself feeling very oncology-like in needing to find hope, in needing to offer some kind of treatment for my desperate patients. I'd find myself confronted with a choice (often an unconscious choice, one I recognize now only in retrospect) between spending the month as a provider of hope (to my patients, to my medical team, and most importantly to myself) or as a dispenser of last rites.

My own emotional needs would shape the way I spoke with my patients. Any surprise that Doug Stevens's doctors had convinced that unfortunate man that his cancer was treatable?

MINISTERS OF HOPE

Rosa Cole had had her tumor removed months earlier, every visible cancer cell cut out of her system by what was no doubt a relentlessly thorough surgeon. And now she sat in her oncologist's office with a tape recorder running on the desk while he explained the troubling images on her latest X-ray and tried his best to put a positive spin on her tragic situation. "Well, you got a tumor that's gonna be, uh, treated with radiation," he told her haltingly. "It's not going to need to be removed. It's going to stay right where—"

"Another tumor?" Cole interjected.

"Huh? Not 'another tumor.' What does another tumor mean?" he replied, a bit confused by the patient's query.

"I thought he cut it out." She hadn't realized that the same tumor, the one that the surgeon had removed so definitively months earlier, hadn't been so definitively removed after all. She was starting to get worried. But the oncologist didn't dwell on the return of the tumor, on its ability to reappear despite all the previous treatments. He emphasized that even now it *could* be treated:

"No, in its position it gets treated with radiation," he explained.

"Benign?" she asked.

What terrible words to hear! The oncologist knew that recurrence of this tumor was a horrible sign that Cole's cancer would be fatal. But Cole still wondered if the tumor was benign? Perhaps wondering now how much reality she could take at once, he tried to reassure her.

"No. It's not. But it's gonna get a good response to radiation," he added, so quickly you wonder if she now realized "it's not benign" meant "it's going to kill you." He continued. "You're gonna get a good response. You're going to be well again. You're going to get a good response."

Talking up hope is an almost unconscious clinical technique for most of us doctors, a technique with a long and noble tradition. The tradition, as we learned earlier, was already firmly established at the time of Hippocrates. The tradition remained strong in the nineteenth century. Thomas Percival, an influential medical ethicist of that era, beseeched his fellow physicians to be "the minister of hope and comfort to the sick." Only with optimistic words, he contended, could the physician "smooth the bed of death . . . and counteract the depressing influence of [their] maladies." The tradition was even made explicit in the AMA's first code of ethics, published in 1847, which admonished physicians "to avoid all things which have a tendency to discourage the patient and to depress his spirits." We even saw that the tradition was running strong as late as the 1960s, when physicians were so committed to being ministers of hope that they withheld cancer diagnoses from their terminally ill patients.

Then came the revolution, and we physicians no longer felt comfortable doling out doses of hope through lies and deception. But that doesn't mean we turned straight from deception to brutal honesty. In my residency, I took care of a patient who had a suspicious mass. The patient was still groggy from the anesthesia, and I was checking out his vital signs when the biopsying surgeon swept through the room. He leaned over the patient to make sure he was awake and blurted out, "It was cancer!" and with almost no other words, left the room. The interaction was so unusual, so awfully awkward and inappropriately blunt, that it has stuck with me to this day. Brutal honesty is not the norm in medical practice; it's not how most of us doctors behave, nor certainly how we strive to behave. We remain Percivalian to this day: Even in the worst situations, we want to give people hope.

And why not? After all, even the most scientific of physicians now recognizes the important role that positive thinking can play in people's health. We recognize it because we've all had experience leveraging the power of the placebo effect.

As the name suggests, the placebo effect refers to the change in health, often the improvement in health, among patients receiving placebos in a clinical trial. Say a group of patients suffer from chronic headaches. Half of the group, chosen at random, receives a new pain pill, and their rate of headaches is cut in half. We know whether this improvement is a result of the new pill by looking at what happens to the placebo group, the other half of the patients who have received an inert "sugar" pill. If their rate of headaches is also cut in half, we can conclude that the pill was ineffective and that their improvement was the result of the placebo effect.

Placebo effects are fueled in part by simple regression to the mean. By the time a person's headaches are so bad that he enrolls in a clinical trial, there's a chance that symptoms will spontaneously improve. But regression to the mean isn't the whole story behind the power of placebos. A substantial part of the placebo effect results instead from mind over matter, from people feeling better simply because they *believe* the pill will make them feel better.

We physicians have seen the power of the placebo in all those trials. We've also seen the power of the placebo in our clinical practice. Not by giving people sugar pills (those pills no longer exist outside of research studies); rather, we add a dose of verbal sugar to the pills we prescribe. When I prescribe a new arthritis pill to one of my patients, for example, I sprinkle my conversation with optimistic anticipations: "Let's take on that knee pain of yours with naproxen. Lots of my patients have told me this pill works better than ibuprofen." I will talk this way to a patient who didn't do well on ibuprofen. I will say the exact opposite to someone who tried naproxen and didn't do well. I'm not lying when I talk this way, because lots of my patients *have* told me that switching from one of these medicines to the other benefited them. These pills, essentially identical in their ability to relieve pain, can provide a benefit due to the placebo effect. A specific patient may feel better because naproxen works better for him than ibuprofen—because of the peculiarities of his biological makeup—or simply because he *believes* it will work better. As a clinician, I'll never know. But I don't care why it works. I'm content knowing that my patient feels better.

Optimistic words are a big part of clinical discourse. Physicians know that such words can make patients feel better. When the neurosurgeon told Mr. Stevens that he could "treat" his cancer, he was trying to help Stevens muster the will to live. He was attempting to bolster Stevens's spirit in advance of what, on the best of days, would be an arduous course of treatment.

Did the neurosurgeon lie to Doug Stevens by saying his cancer was treatable? What about the oncologist who explained to Rosa Cole that the recurrent tumor now visible on her X-ray could be treated with radiation? Did he lie? Eric Cassell, the researcher who tape-recorded that particular encounter, thinks not. In analyzing this encounter, he points out that it took a handful of years for this tumor to end the patient's life, and during most of those years she felt well. But even if it was a lie, writes Cassell, a lie is sometimes still "the best policy." In fact, Cassell counsels physicians that "if they're going to lie, it had better be convincing."

I don't share Cassell's enthusiasm for such deception. And out-and-out lying, like brutal honesty, is the exception among contemporary physicians. Most doctors look for ways to give patients hope without deceiving them. Stevens's cancer, after all, was treatable. So too was Cole's recurrent tumor. Moreover, there is usually enough uncertainty about patient prognoses to find honest ways to communicate hope. So most physicians look for a middle ground, for the hope that lies in the space between realism and deception. One physician described this balancing act to Nicholas Christakis, a physician and sociologist who studies how physicians handle their role as clinical prognosticators. The physician explained that, "Patients will not improve if all hope is denied. Yet it is important to be realistic." Another physician told Christakis, "When patients are terminal, I tell them so in general, nonthreatening terms, and I always leave a ray of hope. But we should not mislead patients."

Aiding physicians in performing this balancing act are stories of miraculous recovery and of unexpected longevity among patients who doctors knew, just *knew* were not long for this world. Most doctors have encountered patients who have survived against all odds. And all have heard about such patients. Their survival tales are the shiny myths that get us through the darkest days of our clinical training.

When I was training at the Mayo Clinic, one of my oncology mentors told me about a terminally ill man he had treated years earlier. The patient had pushed him for prognostic details, wondering how long he had to live. The oncologist, a blunt man by nature, told the patient he was not going to survive more than six months. Angry at this hopeless message, the patient went to another hospital for a last-ditch chemotherapy treatment and (you know where this is going) experienced an unexpectedly good response to it. Six months later, his tumor had not only failed to kill him, but was still in retreat. Having reached the six-month point, he left a phone message for the Mayo oncologist, telling him, "I'm still alive, asshole!"

The oncologist received a series of such profanity-laced messages each year for the next decade, always on the anniversary of the patient's non-death. My mentor told me this story in an effort to persuade me not to repeat his mistake. "Don't hand out death sentences," he told me. "It will only come back to burn you."

In his research, Christakis discovered several stories with close parallels to my mentor's tale. In many versions, the patient is said to outlive the doctor, dancing (at least metaphorically speaking) on the prognosticating physician's grave. The ubiquity of this story—almost always a patient who has been given six months to live—is not necessarily a sign that my mentor's tale was a tall one. Six months is the kind of number doctors would hand out to patients with incurable cancers. Whether true or not, such stories have a huge impact on physician behavior. We start with an instinct to offer hope. Then we learn that on those rare occasions when we are brutally honest with patients, we will be put in our place. Forget the fact that these survival tales contradict our belief that these patients need hope to live. The real moral of the story my mentor told me is, "Don't be a downer! Don't tell dying patients they are dying. No one has anything to gain from that kind of talk."

Plus, such grim prognostication strikes many physicians as being outside their purview. As one physician put it to Christakis, "Saying the situation is hopeless is playing God." Despite the tales of patients outlasting their doctor's stated prognoses, many doctors appear to hold an almost fatalistic view of their communications. Tell a patient he is going to die and somehow you, the doctor, have played too active a role in their end, as if you had doled out a harmful placebo. Physicians can even get snippy in response to prognostic requests. One medical decision-making expert told me about a tape-recorded encounter she listened to in which a spouse pushed a doctor for information about her loved one's prognosis, while the patient muttered in the background about how afraid he was that he was going to die. When the spouse insisted the doctor give them more specific prognostic information, the doctor terminated the conversation by telling her to "try 1-800-Call-God."

In short, the ethic of hope still dominates medical practice, with most physicians shining a bright light on the honest hope that exists in even the most dire circumstances, sometimes to the point that they blind patients to their actual prognoses. Physicians typically do so with the best of intentions, hoping to reduce suffering among their patients. If at all possible, they avoid specific prognostications, fearing not only that, when wrong, such prognostications will be thrown back in their faces, but also that such cold, hard numbers will only add to the cruelty of an already cruel situation.

What happens, then, when physicians are forced to discuss the numbers with their patients?

ANYTHING BUT A BONE MARROW BIOPSY

They had sterilized the skin over William Andrews's hip bone—the posterior iliac crest, for those interested in the specifics—and numbed it up with a local anesthetic, but that didn't mean the procedure had been pain-free. The doctor, you see, had plunged a large needle into the center of Andrews's hip bone, penetrating through the sheath of

nerves and tissues covering the bone, all so he could withdraw precious bone marrow tissue, and that penetration had sent a flurry of
messages racing up to the pain centers in Andrews's brain—holy
mother of what-the-bejeezus!!! Had Andrews known that so many
pain fibers lurked in the recesses of his hip bone, he would have never
allowed the doctors to perform the barbaric procedure, at least not
without first administering general anesthesia. In his five decades of
life, he had never experienced a pain remotely this severe. And the
pain didn't end with the removal of the needle. His hip bone ached
for the better part of a week. Andrews swore then and there that he
would never let a doctor biopsy his bone marrow again.

It would turn out to be a futile promise. A biopsy-free future was
not in the cards for Andrews. After living with a smoldering form of
bone marrow cancer for the previous decade, the former Vegas card
dealer had developed acute leukemia, and if his doctors were to treat
his life-threatening disease, he would need to return for further bone
marrow tissue analysis to monitor his response to therapy.

Andrews was easily the most anxious patient I took care of during
a gray Michigan February when I was working in the hospital caring
for patients admitted to the general medical ward. He had plenty to
be anxious about. His leukemia was raging out of control. His blood
looked like pus, teeming as it was with malignant white blood cells.
At his age—he was almost sixty—and after a decade of chronic bone
marrow cancer, his disease was especially dangerous. Odds were high
that he would not survive another year.

In one of his monologues, Jerry Seinfeld riffs on the idea that
people consider almost nothing to be more scary than death. He starts
by pointing out that people often state that their number one fear is
public speaking, with death coming in as a distant second. "Death
is number two!" Seinfeld exclaims. "Now, this means to the average
person, if you have to go to a funeral, you're better off in the casket
than doing the eulogy." But Andrews wasn't afraid of dying, because
he knew that living in pain can sometimes be worse than passing on

to whatever follows our time on this earth, and he'd already had a firsthand view of death at its worst.

Twenty years earlier, he was living in Vegas and had fallen in love with another card dealer. In the open-minded culture of that city, he had been able to have an out-of-the-closet gay relationship without being judged. He had been truly, ecstatically happy. Nights at the tables, days spent with accepting friends. And his lover, Charles, was simply the best friend he had ever had. "I'd have even loved him," Andrews told me, teary-eyed, "if he'd had a woman's body."

But then Charles got sick, deathly sick. He contracted AIDS at a time when that disease was almost uniformly fatal. Andrews stayed by his side, caring for Charles, ministering to his growing list of bodily needs. He had a ringside seat while his lover wasted away; Charles had been only ninety-five pounds at his death. No bout of leukemia could compare to the suffering Andrews witnessed at his lover's bedside. When Charles died that year, so too did the best part of Andrews's life. He would never fall in love again.

Broken up by the loss of his soul mate, Andrews moved back to rural Michigan, where people weren't so comfortable with his lifestyle. So he became withdrawn. Life didn't mean that much to him anymore. "Don't get me wrong," he said to me. "I'm not suicidal. I don't want to die. It's just that I'm not afraid to die."

It wasn't death, then, that terrified Andrews. It was the thought of another bone marrow biopsy. "You can give me any medicine you want to treat my cancer, but don't—I mean it, don't—ask me to have another bone marrow biopsy."

The decision wasn't mine to make, and not in the new moral paradigm sense of "it's only the patient's decision." No, this was a decision that also relied on the judgment of the consulting oncologist who I had asked to see Andrews. It was the oncology team that had obtained the first bone marrow biopsy and had sent it to the lab for genetic testing, an analysis that would provide crucial information about whether his cancer would respond to treatment. It was they who had the expertise to figure out what course of therapy would maximize his odds of survival and just how important it would be, through a course of such therapy, to obtain further bone marrow samples. Also crucial in determining the relative benefits and burdens of treating his leukemia was prognostication: What chance did he have of gaining long-term survival from treatment (and more importantly to him, from all those subsequent bone marrow biopsies)?

I spoke with the lead oncologist in the hallway outside Andrews's door one day and pushed her for prognostic information. "Best case scenario," she told me, "isn't very promising. If his tumor genetics are favorable, and if he responds well to the chemotherapy, he might have a chance of going into temporary remission. But we won't know the numbers until we get back the genetic analysis."

It took several long days to receive the results, days in which Andrews kept obsessively revisiting the pain of his bone marrow biopsy, and days in which everyone working on my hospital team heard more about Charles's terrible struggle with AIDS. We took turns spending time with Andrews, comforting him, treating any illness-related symptoms. One of the physicians on my team, himself gay, listened for hours to tales of Vegas in the '80s. Then the test results came back, and the oncology team was finally ready to discuss treatment with Andrews. I told them to page me when they were approaching his room so I could listen in on their conversation. When they paged me, I quickly gathered the medical student and the intern and we rushed to his room.

We met the oncology team in the corridor. The news wasn't good, the lead oncologist told me. His tumor genetics revealed—okay, I have to admit the conversation got technical then. Suffice it to say, his tumor didn't have bad genes. It had horrible ones. "Five percent of people with this genetic profile," she told us, "respond to chemotherapy and go into remission." I felt my shoulders sink.

We opened the door to Andrews's room and the oncologist took the lead in discussing treatment options. She explained what the treatment would entail. She compassionately broke the bad news that the genetic tests had not come out well. Andrews was unusually calm. No longer obsessed with bone marrow biopsies, he started asking questions about the chemotherapy. He wondered how many rounds he'd have to go through. She replied that it would depend on how quickly and thoroughly he responded to treatment. He wondered what the odds were of that kind of response. "That is hard to say," the oncologist responded. "The first round of treatment will give us a much better picture."

He told her he knew she couldn't predict the future, but he still wanted to know the odds that he would lick this thing. She paused. These questions are always difficult to answer. And precise numbers? Easy to give a medical colleague a 5 percent figure in the hallway, but here at the bedside, that's much harder. So she took a breath, looked him in the eye, and said, "Twenty percent, Mr. Andrews. We can hope for a twenty percent chance of remission."

"Well, that's a fighting chance," he said, a new light in his eyes. "Let's start treatment."

HOPING FOR HOPE

Twenty percent?! I was stunned. His prognosis had increased fourfold in the three minutes since our hallway conversation. How could this wonderful oncologist, someone I had learned to respect for her compassion and thoughtfulness, have spoken such a blatant falsehood to my nervous patient?

I think she simply panicked. In her left brain—the numbers part of her cerebral cortex—lay the calculations that caused her to derive that 5 percent estimate. Meanwhile, her right brain—the emotional center of her neurologic system—fought back. This man was young-looking for his age, she probably thought to herself. He was such a nervous Nellie too. That low number, delivered under such circumstances, would be negligent in its cruelty. Her brain, I imagine, quickly recalculated his odds in a brief interval of panic, when she realized he was insisting on getting a number out of her.

In July of 1982, Stephen Jay Gould, the famed Harvard paleontologist, was diagnosed with abdominal mesothelioma, a rare cancer that carries a dismal prognosis—so dismal that his doctor (when Gould asked him for suggested readings on the diagnosis) told him to stay away from the library. Gould, of course, ignored this advice and soon discovered that the median length of survival for patients with this diagnosis was a mere eight months.

But Gould would not allow himself to be discouraged by the statistics. As a scientist, he knew that the median was merely a statistical measure, signifying that half the patients lived this long and half did not. So, which half would he be in? From his reading, he knew he was younger and healthier than the typical mesothelioma patient. Right there he was confident: He would live more than eight months. His mathematical reasoning now in high gear, no doubt nudged along by very motivated reasoning elsewhere in his brain, Gould soon convinced himself that he would be a long-term survivor, a conclusion that would prove to be accurate. He died twenty years later of an unrelated cancer.

I expect that Andrews's oncologist that day, when pressed by her nervous patient, did a Gouldian recalculation of her own. Maybe she convinced herself that Andrews was younger or healthier than the average leukemia patient, or that somehow the genetic test wasn't as predictive in his case as in others. Doctors, it turns out, are prey to all kinds of unrealistically optimistic impulses. Christakis uncovered widespread optimism in his studies of physicians' prognostications. In one survey, he asked doctors to predict how long their specific patients would live, patients who were terminally ill at the time of the study. He discovered that doctors systematically overestimated their patients' life expectancy. If a physician predicted his patient would live for four months, odds were the patient would live closer to two or three months.

Why such dismal prognostications among physicians intimately familiar with their patients' medical situations? Perhaps they are so motivated to find hope that they convince themselves their patients have weeks, even months to live, even though those same patients would end up living for only days or weeks. Such miscalculations undoubtedly contribute to delays in referring patients to hospice care. Many patients only embrace hospice care and all the comforts such care can provide in the very last days of their lives. Many would benefit from earlier referral to hospice, but hope stands in the way of timeliness.

Such unrealistic optimism wasn't the problem with Andrews that day, however. After all, the oncologist had been quite willing to deliver a grim prognosis to me in the hallway. It was only when she spoke with Andrews that the prognosis had turned relatively rosy. Yet her behavior that day, the sudden switch from 5 percent to 20 percent, is another common phenomenon shaping communication between doctors and patients near the end of life. On top of being overly optimistic about how long their patients will live, most physicians still communicate an even rosier prediction to their patients. Ask a doctor how long his patient will live and he'll tell his colleagues one number—perhaps, four months—and communicate an even better number to his patient—six or eight months—even though the truth is closer to two or three months. In painting this overly optimistic picture to their patients, I'd have to guess that the doctors simply find it too painful to tell the truth, even to themselves. Under the new paradigm, it seems as if out-and-out lies are out, but exaggerations—what more generously might be called generous interpretations—are in.

THE CONSEQUENCES OF EXAGGERATION

As I left Andrews's room that day, still stunned at the 20 percent figure handed to him by the oncologist, I knew I couldn't let him undergo treatment in the face of such misinformation. So the intern and I returned to his room to find out what treatment was really in his best interests. I pulled up a chair and sat across from Andrews, who was sitting sideways on his bed, stooped over with his feet touching the floor. I asked him what he thought the treatment would feel like.

"It'll make me feel like crap," he replied. I asked him if he realized that they'd monitor his response to treatment by repeating the bone marrow biopsy. "I know, Dr. Ubel, I know. Just give me strong meds, please," he pleaded. I expressed some surprise at his change of attitude toward the biopsy.

"But, Doctor," he said, "Charles would want me to fight. That wonderful man . . . he fought to the bitter end. Don't you think he would want me to do the same?"

"I think he'd want whatever made you happy. But I'm trying to make sure I understand what you're saying. If the treatment had only a one in a hundred chance of prolonging your life?" I asked.

"I'd still try. I owe it to Charles."

I walked out of the room confident that the 20 percent figure hadn't been the key thing influencing his choice. I wouldn't have chosen to undergo treatment in his situation, or so I believed at the time, but I saw no reason to persuade him otherwise.

Not all prognostic miscommunications can be so readily addressed. Consider Doug Stevens, the man I discussed at the beginning of this chapter whose cancer, he was told, couldn't be cured but could nevertheless be treated. By the time he arrived under my care, his lung cancer had been blasted with radiation and targeted with powerful drugs. The tumors in his brain had been removed by the very neurosurgeon whose confidence in the treatability of his disease had launched Stevens down this path. The cancer in his lungs had continued to grow over the past months, despite all the treatment, to the point that it was now causing the pneumonia that would hasten his death. But the hastening was being held off by hope. Stevens and his family decided over the next several days to undergo every possible treatment, even as the burden of these treatments grew.

The pneumonia was no simple bacterial infection, but we didn't know that right away. So the antibiotics we gave Stevens upon admission were ineffective against the invading organism and only had the effect of causing terrible diarrhea, a doubly bad side effect for Stevens given that he was too weak to make it to the bathroom quickly enough to keep up with the movement of his bowels. So we "diapered him up" and began monitoring him for pressure ulcers on his sacrum, recognizing that the combination of fecal incontinence and being bedridden would put his skin at considerable risk for damage.

Is this the best way for Stevens to spend the last days of his life, I wondered? I returned to his bedside each day and readdressed the goals of treatment, explaining that his tumor was fatal. "It is going to kill you," I'd say. "We can't do anything to stop that." He would express his understanding but . . . there would always be a "but": but could I talk to his sister, could I ask the neurosurgeon to talk to his sister, could I wait and see what happened after another few days of treatment.

When we figured out that his lung infection was fungal, we switched therapies, but his fungal infection had already spread enough that it caused another problem: He became increasingly somnolent and confused. The fungus had spread to the lining of his brain and was blocking off the flow of fluid around his head and spinal cord, thereby increasing the pressure in this fluid cavity and, essentially, squashing his brain.

As he drifted away from us, I instructed our team to aggressively promote his comfort. The last few days had arrived, I thought, and I wanted those days to be free of suffering. But that afternoon I was paged by the infectious-disease team. "Why haven't you arranged for an urgent spinal tap?" they asked me. The infection was treatable, they told me, and he would die from intracranial pressure before the antifungals took hold unless I performed a spinal tap. Stevens's sister received an update on the situation by telephone and quickly got hold of the neurosurgeon, whom she had come to trust back in the days when he was sprinkling their world with hope dust. The neurosurgeon also called me up, frantic that I do the procedure.

We conducted the spinal tap that evening, and by the next morning Stevens was beginning to become more coherent. I spoke with him then. He had already talked with his sister. He wanted me to treat his fungal infection with "everything you've got."

Over the next few days, we gained ground on his fungal infection, all the while aware that Stevens's tumor was advancing. Then he developed a terrible rash, with itching so severe that he became delirious from lack of sleep. We treated the symptoms of his rash, a rash caused either by his antifungal treatment or by one of his dozen other medications, but he continued to waste away as the combination of infection and tumor raised his metabolic rate well beyond his ability to ingest calories.

Stevens died two weeks later. His last few days were ones of comfort and peace, but most of those two weeks preceding the final hours were far from comfortable or peaceful. The ethic of hope—of building up this man's spirits—combined with a culture of aggressive treatment ("the standard of care for such fungal infections is to perform regular spinal taps!") conspired to prolong his suffering. Conspired with the help of one other factor too: Stevens's own desire to pursue hope beyond reason.

MOVED TO ACT

It was an admittedly artificial choice, but one that Jonathan Baron, a decision psychologist at the University of Pennsylvania, constructed to reveal the psychological forces underlying people's decisions. He asked people to imagine that a virulent flu was coming to town, universally fatal to whoever contracted it, with experts estimating that a full 10 percent of the population would be infected. Fortunately, a vaccine was available that would prevent infection. But there was one caveat: 5 percent of people would have a fatal reaction to the vaccine—the vaccine that was supposed to save their lives would instead kill them. A straightforward choice, then: a 10 percent risk of death from the flu versus a 5 percent risk of death from the vaccine. What would you do?

As it turns out, a sizable minority of people said that they would forgo the vaccine, preferring to face a higher risk of death from the flu and avoiding taking an action that could cause their death. For these people, the harms of omission, or inaction, are preferred to the harms of commission, or action.

For all its artificiality, Baron's hypothetical choice has received lots of attention in the medical decision-making community because it captures an important phenomenon. Many people *do* refuse vaccines when they learn that the vaccines carry serious side effects, even when the chances of experiencing such side effects are significantly less than the odds of benefiting from the vaccine. This scenario also captures the general paranoia many people feel about vaccines. Many people believe, for instance, that vaccines cause autism, despite a wealth of evidence to the contrary. Michele Bachmann, when campaigning in the Republican presidential primaries in 2011, even believed it when one of her supporters told her that the HPV vaccine had caused her adolescent daughter to become "mentally retarded." No wonder, then, that at the first hint of trouble, many people avoid the flu vaccine like the plague.

But is this preference to inaction limited to stigmatized interventions like vaccines? To find an answer to this question, I presented people with a variation of this flu-shot scenario. In the first variation, I asked people to imagine that they had been diagnosed with a slow-growing cancer and, if they chose to leave the cancer untreated for the

moment—if they chose a strategy of watchful waiting, monitoring
the cancer and only treating it if it showed signs of spreading—they
would experience a 10 percent lifetime risk of dying from the cancer.
Alternatively, I explained that they could treat the cancer right away
with chemotherapy. The chemotherapy would cure the cancer but,
like the flu vaccine described in Baron's original scenario, it carried a
risk of death: 5 percent of people receiving the chemotherapy would
die as a result of the treatment. Once again, a straightforward choice:
do nothing and face a 10 percent chance of death, or do something
and face a 5 percent chance of death from treatment.

Despite the similar structure of these decisions, when it came to
cancer and chemotherapy, almost *no one* said they would forgo the
treatment. People preferred action to inaction. People are more willing
to accept treatment complications when imagining cancer treatment
than when contemplating flu vaccines. But how much more willing?

I posed a revised version of this choice to another group of people.
In this scenario, I asked people to imagine that watchful waiting led
to only a 5 percent chance of death from the cancer whereas surgery,
which would cure the cancer, carried a 10 percent risk of death. In
this case, a substantial majority of people said they wanted the surgery, preferring death from activity to death from inactivity. "Get it
out of me," they said. "Better to go out fighting than to wait for bad
things to happen." The thought of untreated cancer bothered these
people so much that they preferred taking action, even when that
action was more likely to harm them.

Sometimes even artificial choices reveal fundamental truths about
human nature. In this case, people's choices jibed with what I had
seen so many times in real life. Cancer, "the big C," creates a powerful
compulsion to act. I have witnessed this phenomenon dozens of times
among older men with localized prostate cancer for whom surgery has
not been shown to yield any survival advantages, but who nevertheless
opt for this treatment, willing to put up with impotence and inconti-

nence just to know that they have done everything in their power to "kill the beast," as one patient put it to me.

A strong psychological call to action, then, compels many patients to opt for arduous treatments in the face of life-threatening diagnoses like cancer. Another psychological force influences patients in these same situations, that instinct we saw earlier exhibited by Stephen Jay Gould: to convince themselves that the odds of survival are better than those of the average patient afflicted with the same disease. In Gould's case, he was right to view himself as better than average. He was a fine scientist with a good knowledge of statistics, and his optimism largely derived from data-based reasoning. The vast majority of patients share his optimism, despite lacking any scientific reason to do so. And last I checked, it's impossible for everyone to be above average. Yet if a doctor tells a patient he has no more than six months to live, or no more than a 10 percent chance of responding to treatment, most patients immediately ratchet up the numbers. Six months becomes nine; 10 percent becomes 20 percent. The ratcheting occurs at the speed of a brain stem reflex.

Given these powerful psychological phenomena, is it any wonder that physicians offer patients so much last-ditch chemotherapy, so many troublingly toxic treatments, treatments that cause predictable suffering yet bring only the slightest chance of benefit? Motivated by an unconscious desire for optimism, they overestimate patients' chances of survival. Moved by the difficulty of giving people bad news, they then present even more exaggerated prognoses to their patients. Patients respond, of course, by inflating these estimates even more and then wed these inflated estimates to their need for action. A patient with a 10 percent chance of survival is believed to have a 15 or 20 percent chance by his physician, who communicates an even better prognosis to the patient—maybe 25 percent, 35 percent—and now that patient convinces himself he'll do even better. Voilà! The universal desire for hope has created a psychology of immortality.

THE STATE OF THE REVOLUTION

The patient-empowerment revolution was launched by people fighting back against doctors who insisted on keeping patients alive against their wishes. While the revolution has enabled patients and their families to set limits—to tell doctors it's time to stop—and while in its most radical form the revolution has even led to the legalization of physician-assisted suicide in some locations, the revolution can't overcome the psychology of terminal illness. Quite often the need for hope and the desire for action causes doctors and patients to pursue what are essentially futile measures. As a result, close to 40 percent of Medicare spending in the United States occurs in the last six months of people's lives. Few experts think that all of this spending and all of these medical interventions are promoting patients' best interests.

If you desire a measure of where things stand and of how successful the shared decision-making revolution has been at getting patients the right amount of health care, you need look no further than end-of-life decision making. All the problems we have seen over the previous few chapters are on display at the end of life. The problems created by physician jargon? Not only on display ("We can treat your cancer") but also particularly influential, because as the end of life approaches, patients become even more inclined to misinterpret their physicians' words in ways that will provide them with hope. The failure of doctors and patients to recognize and respond to each other's emotions? Also on display in uniquely powerful forms. The end of life often brings out strong negative emotions, in both doctors and patients—the very kind of emotions each party has the greatest difficulty communicating to the other. The unconscious psychological factors influencing people's decisions? On display inarguably in their strongest form.

Even though the revolution began in large part at the bedsides of dying patients, the state of medical decision making at the end of life is frankly dismal. The revolution has so far failed to achieve its goals. The patient-empowerment revolution rose up over the previous few decades so that patients would receive medical care that promotes their best interests, and of course so they don't receive medical care that works against their best interests. But by that measure, the revolution has failed. It has transformed the way doctors and patients talk to each other, but not in a manner that promotes good decision making. The revolution is like a shiny new car without functioning parts. It looks beautiful, but when you sit down inside it, the car won't take you where you want to go.

But there's a way to move this car down the road. We simply need a new engine. Instead of relying on informed patients to power the revolution on their own, we need to teach patients how to partner with their physicians. We need a revolution centered on the idea of shared decision making.

PART III

From Empowerment to Partnership

EIGHT
Getting Good Advice

Isaac Palmer lay in his hospital bed at the Mayo Clinic only remotely aware of his surroundings, a wide range of colon cancer metastases having thrown his metabolic functions into disarray. I spoke with his two children, explaining that his cancer was incurable. Because they were his next of kin, I told them they would be responsible for deciding which interventions their father would receive, as long as he remained too confused to decide for himself. We spoke for a few minutes about his dire situation, a conversation that went as well as can be expected given the difficult topic at hand. (It is never easy to tell anyone that their dad is dying.) Then I turned the conversation toward an even more difficult topic. As the medical resident caring for Mr. Palmer, it was my job to discuss his DNR status, to determine whether his children were in favor of a Do Not Resuscitate order.

The medical literature had taught me that metastatic cancer and cardiopulmonary resuscitation (CPR) were a dismal combination. Generally, when patients with metastatic cancer experience cardiac arrests—when their hearts stop—almost nothing can bring them back to life, meaning the patients will die despite the frantic, sleep-deprived efforts of the code team. Moreover, in those rare cases when CPR does restart these patients' hearts, they still aren't likely to survive their hospital stays, because their cardiopulmonary systems inevitably shut down again as their cancers progress. My goal, then, in discussing CPR with Palmer's two children was to help them understand its futility, so they would endorse a DNR order, thereby saving all of us from putting him through the horrors of a "code red."

I struck a pedagogical pose and described the situation. "Your father's cancer is incurable," I explained. "We have no more chemo to offer. And even though we'll try to treat his kidney problem, he may be too sick to recover." They nodded their heads in sorrowful acknowledgment while I continued doling out bad news. "And if your dad's illness progresses, and his heart and lungs stop working, I don't think he'd survive resuscitation."

"We understand," said his son. His daughter remained mute, but between dabs of her handkerchief, she nodded yes to her brother's pronouncement. I was confident now that I'd accurately informed them of the situation and that the time was right to ask them to make a decision.

"So," I continued, "if his heart stops, would you want us to try to restart it?"

Their body language suddenly changed. I was no longer simply informing them about their dad; I was now soliciting their opinion about his care. "What are you asking, Doctor?" said his son.

"I'm asking whether you want your dad to be DNR, meaning that if his heart stops, we will not try to restart it with CPR."

"Well, I don't want Dad to die," his daughter blurted out, distressed now with the direction of the conversation.

"Of course you don't," I said as compassionately as possible. "I'm just asking whether, if he *does* die—I mean if his heart and lungs stop working." (I was beginning to panic now, having lost control of this delicate conversation.) "Would you be okay with us not trying to bring him back to life?"

"Oh, no. You can't abandon him," the son replied.

As we saw in the previous chapter, end-of-life decisions often create a psychology of desperation, causing doctors, patients, and even their families to hope beyond hope. But hope wasn't the issue here. This family knew their dad was going to die soon, and they understood that he wouldn't survive CPR. Yet they couldn't sign off on a DNR order, because they were overwhelmed by the thought that doing so would amount to killing him.

In accordance with the new paradigm, I had patiently educated this family about the facts relevant to their father's care, but our conversation had ground to a halt because they couldn't do what they knew they needed to do—they couldn't make their father DNR even though they knew their decision could cause him to suffer.

It was the late 1980s, and by this point in my training I had already held countless DNR conversations. Some of the families I had spoken with were ready to set limits, to make their loved ones DNR, even to limit other aggressive and futile treatments. But more often the families panicked at the thought of a DNR order, unwilling to be the ones responsible for their loved one's death.

Worried that the Palmer children would panic that day, I switched tactics. "If your father's heart stops," I told them forcefully, "we would have to pound on his chest to try to restart it and jam a tube down his throat to restart his lungs." I gestured adamantly in unison with each shocking verb. "We'd need to stab needles into his arteries and force thousands of volts of electricity through his breastbone. As sick as he is, our chest pounding will probably break some of his ribs. And if he survives this treatment, he'll have to go to the ICU where he'll probably spend the last few days of his life, surrounded by IV tubes and medical machinery. Is that really what you want for your dad?"

With graphic language like this, I had taken the moral ideals of autonomy and twisted them to my own ends. Consistent with the new paradigm, I hadn't withheld information from my patient's family. I'd very well bludgeoned them with information. Every word I had told them was true, but I had chosen the kind of emotive language guaranteed to get them in line.

I'm ashamed of the way I acted that day. A family had arrived in the hospital, terrified about what was happening to their father, and I had assaulted them with violent verbiage. No doubt put off by my bludgeoning, the Palmer children refused to make him DNR. And who could blame them? They'd only met me minutes earlier and here I was asking them, practically forcing them, to sign his death sentence.

And all the while, there was a better way I could have handled things that day, a way to turn this confrontational conversation into a true partnership.

FIRST UNDERSTANDING, THEN ADVICE

Allison Hall had suffered her first stroke a half-dozen years earlier, with several ministrokes following like aftershocks. She had lived in a nursing home for several years, slowly losing her ability to function. On a good day twelve months earlier, she might have recognized her oldest daughter. But now she returned her daughter's smiles with a vacant stare.

It was the mid-1990s, and I was a relatively new faculty member at the University of Pennsylvania. My hospital team had spoken with Hall's three children on the morning of admission, to determine how much of her current condition was acute versus chronic. She had a urinary tract infection, the kind of illness that often makes mildly demented patients appear to be severely demented. The fever and accompanying metabolic disarray stresses out a brain that is already teetering on the edge of cognitive dysfunction. Before making important decisions about her care, we first needed to understand what her life would be like once her acute problem was under control. From what we learned, it became clear that Hall had lost track of reality long ago, well before this infection. She was "pleasantly demented"— happy most of the time, even though she kept mistaking her granddaughter for her oldest child.

As the senior physician in charge of the case, I was not the person who would normally discuss DNR orders with the family. That job was normally left to the medical resident or intern. But by then I had found a better way to hold such conversations, and I often took the lead in at least one such interaction early in the month so the trainees could see my approach. (Medical teaching often follows the "see one, do one, teach one" approach, so I had to contribute by giving them one to see.)

I didn't expect Mrs. Hall to experience a cardiac arrest during this hospital stay, but I still felt it was important to discuss CPR with her family should things take a turn for the worse. I began by talking with her kids about their goals. I asked them what they hoped to accomplish during this hospital stay. They were unanimous in their desire for their mom to return to the nursing home, but not at any and all cost. More than anything, they wanted their mom to be happy.

"We can help with that," I said. "We can treat this infection and see if it turns around. But if it doesn't, if she's too frail to bounce back, we can make sure we stick with the kinds of medical care that will make her feel better and avoid the kinds that will make her miserable." They told me that such an approach was just what they wanted for their mom.

I then laid out what we would do to improve her quality of life. I explained that I would ask the nursing staff to let their mom sleep through the night without unnecessary blood draws and vital-sign checks. (In demented patients, sleep interruptions can lead to agitation and delirium.) I informed them that we would treat her with antibiotics to try to cure the infection, so she wouldn't suffer from fevers any longer. I told them we'd give her medicines to combat her fever in the meantime. And, finally, I said we would test her regularly for any signs of pain or discomfort and aggressively treat those symptoms.

Then I redirected the conversation from what we'd *do* for her to what we might *not* do—to deciding whether to make her DNR. Only this time I didn't throw the decision in their faces ("Do you want to make your mom DNR?"). Nor did I assault them with graphic verbiage. I folded the DNR discussion into a larger conversation about their goals for her hospital stay: "As we've discussed, we're all determined to make your mom as comfortable as possible. So I think it makes great sense to try these antibiotics and other medicines to see if they improve the way she is feeling, maybe even help her get back to the nursing home. But if her heart stops, or if she goes into respiratory failure—if she no longer has the ability to breathe on her own—if those things happen, I don't think we should do CPR or put her on the ventilator in the ICU. As frail as she is, she would have a hard time making it through such interventions. And as confused as she is, she might end up experiencing pain without understanding what we are trying to do to her. If things get so bad that her heart stops, I would like to make her comfortable, but I would not recommend any of those more aggressive measures. Does that sound right to you?"

After my residency at the Mayo, when I had tried to bludgeon families into DNR orders, I discovered behavioral economics, which taught me to think carefully about how I framed choices to patients and families. In this case, I framed the conversation in terms of a recommendation, one that I gave the family only after understanding their goals. I had by then taken this approach a number of times, usually with great success, though success was not measured by whether they accepted my recommendation. In fact, some families resisted my recommendation. In those cases, I never responded with chest-pounding, needle-jabbing language. Resuscitating a dying patient is not the worst thing we doctors can do. Making a family regret their decision is far worse. However, in the vast majority of these conversations, my recommendation was met not with resistance but relief. They didn't want their loved one to suffer, and they knew that CPR would only prolong their pain. But they didn't want to be the ones who made that choice. My recommendation helped them by sharing the decision-making burden.

Making recommendations has long been a part of medical practice.

But ever since the rise of patient self-determination, physicians have struggled to know when or whether to provide recommendations to their patients. Some physicians are quite comfortable dispensing advice, doling out recommendations like Halloween candy. Other physicians believe that respecting patient autonomy requires them to forgo recommendations, even when their patients request advice. I have come across this belief many times when listening to encounters between doctors and patients. In many encounters, patients ask for advice only to meet stiff resistance. "That's not my decision to make," the physician will say, as if chanting an inviolable moral mantra.

The profession's ambivalence toward recommendations is understandable. On one hand, many patients and families have come to depend on doctors for advice. On the other hand, recommendations can easily become coercive. The distinction between "you need surgery" and "I recommend you get surgery" can be quite subtle.

Like physicians, patients hold a wide range of views about physician recommendations. Some patients behave as if they have no need for doctorly advice, arriving at their appointments armed with research, convinced they have already figured out their own diagnosis and treatment. The lack of a medical license is the only thing preventing them from prescribing their own therapy. Others don't want a thing to do with their medical decisions, expecting their doctor to relieve them of all difficult choices. Of course, many change their view of physician recommendations depending on the circumstances, perhaps relying on their doctors to decide which blood pressure medicine is best but adamant that they see an orthopedic surgeon for their knee pain rather than a physical therapist.

What I'm trying to say is that the proper role of physician recommendations in medical decision making is complicated. Nevertheless, delving into this complex topic is the best way for us to begin to see how to move from patient empowerment to a doctor–patient partnership. Physician recommendations, when handled well, are a paradigm of shared decision making. But when handled poorly, they are the proverbial wolf in sheep's clothing: paternalism disguised as advice.

An understanding of physician recommendations—more specifically, of the psychological factors that influence the giving and taking of medical advice—will show us the steps doctors and patients need to take in order to create an environment in which informed and empowered patients meet up with physicians who are ready and able to partner with them.

THE FEEL OF RESPONSIBILITY

When Tracy Malloy visited her gynecologist for her annual exam, she felt as if she were in the early stages of a minor cold. But she quickly took a turn for the worse and two days later called the gynecologist back up. Soon, she found herself in a bed at the Women's and Children's Hospital with a fever that would have made her miserable if it hadn't been overwhelmed by the worst headache of her life. The hospital doctor ordered some tests and gave her Tylenol. "But he didn't give her emergency antibiotics," the resident told me. "Can you believe it?"

The question was rhetorical. Malloy had been transferred from the Women's and Children's Hospital (an institution primarily designed to care for obstetric and gynecologic conditions) to the university hospital where I worked at the time because her condition was deteriorating rapidly. I was the senior physician, and the medical resident had begun telling me Malloy's story. "The patient," he said in near disbelief, "had clear signs of neck stiffness but sat around at the Women's hospital while the doctor waited for tests . . . and they didn't even get an LP [a spinal tap] for another hour!" The resident was shocked because the Women's hospital had failed to diagnose the patient's bacterial meningitis in a timely manner.

Internal specialists like me are trained to be paranoid about bacterial meningitis. A routine-looking upper-respiratory infection can rapidly devolve into a life-threatening illness if the invading organism thrives on devouring neurologic tissue. The meningococcal bacteria, for instance, usually live harmlessly inside healthy people, minding their own business. But for reasons not fully understood, the bacteria can metamorphose from peaceful to dangerous in a matter of days. A headache, fever, and stiff neck—symptoms that often signal the arrival of a bad cold—can also be the first signs that the meningococcus has found its way into the meninges, the soft tissue covering the brain and spinal cord, where it will reproduce rapidly and dangerously. If a patient's neck is suspiciously stiff, and if she gets a certain kind of fearful look on her face, we internists worry about bacterial meningitis. In such situations, the mantra is "treat now, diagnose later." Get powerful antibiotics in a patient's system right away and then, only then, establish the diagnosis with an LP.

Unfortunately, such paranoia was lacking that day in the Women's hospital. The doctors hadn't started antibiotics on this patient, waiting instead for her test results to come back; in the meantime, the infection had marched through her body like an invading army. By the time she was emergently transferred to our hospital, she had already suffered permanent hearing loss. Everyone on my team was astonished at the negligence of the outside physicians. The entire team felt that someone, some "power that be," needed to take action against these physicians. "The patient needs to find a lawyer, pronto," said one intern. "The state medical licensing board needs to investigate too," the resident added.

Impressed by their passion, I introduced a few questions to probe the strength of their convictions. "Are you going to tell the patient about your concerns?" I asked. They began backpedaling furiously. "It's not my job to initiate lawsuits," the resident replied. "What about the medical board?" I wondered. "Will you notify them about your concerns? How about the administrators at the Women's hospital?"

With responsibility now placed on their shoulders, their confidence was suddenly shattered. "We weren't there when she presented to the Women's hospital," the resident said. "Maybe her exam wasn't so obvious then." One of the interns followed up with a story about one of his patients who had an unusual presentation of the same disease.

In asking those questions, I had intended to discuss the ethics of the situation with the medical team, exploring our duties as physicians to regulate our profession. However, as so often happens when I explore ethics, I found myself surrounded by psychology. On the surface, the psychology looked pretty simplistic and, frankly, unethical. These young doctors were psychologically resistant to "tattling" on their colleagues, the social psychology of kindergarten tribesmanship overcoming their moral duties. But as a new attending physician, one who had been a resident himself only months previously, I was aware of another powerful psychological force exerting itself that day. I knew from my own experience that decisions feel very different when you become the final decision maker, when you become the "here" in the "the buck stops here."

As a resident the previous year, I had cared for a patient with a life-threatening disease, with no proven therapy available to stave off his inevitable demise. The attending physician prescribed an unproven and expensive therapy, and I leapt into rhetorical action, pointing out the potential harms of the treatment. I even reminded the attending how quickly medical costs are rising. The only effect of my diatribe was to lower my grade for the rotation. In another case that month I had cared for someone with pneumonia who had responded well to treatment. I told the attending that I thought the patient was ready to go home, only to be rebuffed: "We need to watch the patient in the hospital for one more night and make sure his white count normalizes." I was irate at what I considered a lame decision. I deemed it overcautious and expensive, and I promised myself that, when I was an attending, I wouldn't be so weak.

And then, of course, I became an attending and found myself on the other end of the same conversation. "He's improving nicely. He should do fine at home," the resident would tell me. A rush of anxiety would pass through me. *He could easily take a turn for the worse,* I'd think, *and even though his white blood cell count is improving, it isn't yet normal.* It was no longer easy to be cavalier and send the patient home.

Being responsible for decisions changes judgment. Indeed, it was sometime after becoming an attending physician—a responsible decision maker—that I figured out why so many of my earlier end-of-life conversations had gone so terribly wrong. I had entered into these conversations with patients or their families believing that clinical facts would rule the day—the prognostications, the pros and cons of CPR. I had held the same belief when arguing with my attending physicians about the proper way to care for our patients. I had thought that the attendings disagreed with me because they were behind on the literature, blind to the facts. But those families I "counseled" on end-of-life care and those attending physicians I "lectured" on medical evidence were making different decisions than I was not because they believed different facts but because they were responsible for the consequences of their choices.

It was only when I finished my training and became the clinical decision maker of last resort that I realized the impact responsibility can have on decision making. All those families who couldn't designate their loved ones as DNR, it was their overwhelming sense of responsibility that was pushing them away from the best choice.

ASSUMING THE BURDEN

When the supreme court of New Jersey granted Joe Quinlan the right to control his daughter Karen's destiny, Joe's sense of relief at winning the case was soon joined by an even stronger emotion: the burden of responsibility. He felt the crushing weight of the decision now bearing down on him. "I had the final say," he said to a reporter writing about Karen's story, "and that, to me, was an awful responsibility. Being the final judge." So he sought out someone who would relieve him of this burden. "I knew I really needed to talk to Father Tom."

He sat down with his pastor, Father Tom, and laid out his anxieties. "I have the final say," he told Father Tom, "and this decision bothers me something terrible. Am I playing God?"

"Don't worry that you're making a decision in Karen's death," Father Tom replied. "God has made the decision that she's going to die. You're just agreeing with God's decision, that's all."

Father Tom demonstrated great wisdom that day in partnering Joe with God—a beautiful way of helping Joe come to terms with his own choice. No longer did Joe feel like the sole decision maker deciding Karen's fate. He didn't have to wonder whether he had played God. God was playing God; Joe was simply accepting God's advice.

Father Tom's strategy is a good analogy for the way a physician's recommendation can relieve patients and families of the burden of making difficult decisions on their own. When a physician recommends a course of action, the patient is no longer alone in choosing that particular path. When I spoke with Allison Hall's family and recommended that we not resuscitate their ill mother, I relieved them of the burden of playing God. After loved ones die, many families suffer for months with the feeling that they were at fault for the way things ended. Medical researchers have even documented post-traumatic stress disorder among survivors, with one such survivor poignantly telling the research team, "The thing I loved most in my life I didn't want to kill. That's the part I agonized over a lot."

When physicians make recommendations, they relieve patients and families of the burden of responsibility. Patients are thus no longer alone in making the decision, no longer playing God. They are simply deciding whether to take the doctor's advice.

I recognize the risk of taking Father Tom's clever idea of following God's advice and twisting it so that a physician, in effect, plays the role of God. No doubt, physicians need to offer recommendations with humility and in a manner that invites divergence of opinion. As I will show later, physicians must be cautious in offering recommendations to patients, if for no other reason than the strong influence such recommendations can have on patients' choices. But there are other reasons for caution. Chief among them, the strange way in which the very act of making a recommendation alters how people weigh the pros and cons of decisions.

RECOMMEND UNTO OTHERS

An attractive stranger from across a crowded room keeps looking your way. You have even made eye contact. And now you have to decide: Should you go up and introduce yourself? The stakes are clear. Introduce yourself and you will experience anxiety ("What should I say? Should I play hard to get or just act natural?") and face the prospect of rejection. However, if things go well, you might make a new friend, maybe even start a life-changing romantic relationship! A rational weighing of the pros and cons points you in but one direction—the benefits of making a love connection far outweigh the short-term pain of rejection. But you take a swig of your drink and continue conversing with your friends, too scared to take the risk.

Now, suppose the situation is slightly different. Same bar, same friends, same attractive stranger seated across the room—yet this time the stranger is glancing not at you but at your friend. And your friend is glancing back, struggling to decide whether to say hello. Your friend leans in and asks for your advice. "Should I go up and say hi?" Is there any doubt what you would recommend? Is there any question that you'd tell your friend to go for it? After all, what's the worst thing that could happen—they'll feel bad for half a beer?

Giving advice changes the feel of decisions, sometimes in ways that improve decision making. In the case of barstool decision making, when people give advice to friends they are less swayed by the fear of short-term pain of social rejection from a pickup line gone bad. Short-term fear can push people away from choices that yield the best chance of long-term happiness.

When researchers have asked people to identify decisions they regret from their past, people typically don't recall actions they took that didn't work out well. Instead, they kick themselves over actions they *didn't* take. They regret not asking Amy out before she met that triathlete (purely hypothetical example, of course). They wish they had volunteered for that job in Africa. They wish they'd taken a few more risks and hadn't chickened out of so many of life's opportunities.

I expect that many of these inactions would not have happened if people had solicited advice from their friends. Consider a study conducted by two experts in decision psychology, Laura Kray and Rich Gonzalez. Kray and Gonzalez asked college students to imagine that they had just graduated from college and had two job offers in hand. The first offer carries with it a great chance for wealth and prestige. The second offer consists of more modest pay but a much greater chance for self-fulfillment and a real opportunity to benefit humanity. Kray and Gonzalez found that students were significantly more likely to recommend the second job, the one with lower pay and greater fulfillment, to a friend than they were to choose it for themselves.

The same phenomenon reveals itself when people make medical decisions. Consider the colon cancer decision I wrote about in chapter 6, the one that presented a trade-off between death and unpleasant side effects such as wound infections or colostomies. When I posed this hypothetical scenario to a national sample of primary care physicians in the United States, a staggering 40 percent of them were so put off by the unpleasant side effects—even temporary ones, like slow-healing wound infections—that they opted for the alternative, which increased their odds of dying from colon cancer. But my survey didn't end with this one group of physicians. I asked another group of physicians what treatment they would recommend if one of their *patients* were diagnosed with the same illness—the same decision, the same exact trade-off, except now physicians were advice givers. With this altered mind-set, the vast majority of physicians recommended that patients choose the survival-maximizing treatment, explaining in the margins of my survey that it was better to live with these side effects than to die of colon cancer. Despite being desensitized to things like bodily functions, physicians are (almost) as human as anyone else, influenced by emotions and psychological forces to make choices that don't promote their best interests. Yet when put in the role of advice giver, physicians are less susceptible to these same emotions.

When doctors shift roles from decision maker to advice giver, their thinking changes. And they are largely unaware of the change. When I asked these same doctors whether they would recommend a different treatment to patients than what they would choose for themselves, almost all said no. They didn't realize that the framing of the question ("What would you do?" versus "What would you recommend?") would influence their thinking. The psychology of advice giving lies hidden beneath conscious awareness.

Ask "What should I do, Doc?" and you might get a different answer than if you ask "What would you do, Doc?" Ask "What would you do if it was your mother?" and you may get different advice than if you ask "What do you think is best for *my* mother?" Getting confused yet?

WARNING: RECOMMENDATIONS ARE DANGEROUSLY INFLUENTIAL!

What I've covered so far in this chapter might look like an unequivocal endorsement of physician recommendations. I've explained how recommendations relieve patients and families from the responsibility of making decisions on their own. I've described experiments establishing that making recommendations changes the way people think, helping them to avoid psychological forces known to otherwise bias their decisions. But there is a dark side to recommendations. For starters, recommendations influence patients to choose treatments that they would otherwise avoid. For example, suppose you have to decide whether to get vaccinated against a new strain of the flu. In addition, imagine that the vaccine causes more harm than it provides benefits. If you are like most people, you will not go for the vaccine . . . unless I also happen to tell you that your doctor recommends the vaccine.

I ran an experiment in which I described this hypothetical vaccine to people. I told them about its risks and benefits in language so plain that almost everyone could see that the vaccine was not a good idea. But with half of the people I surveyed, I also told them two additional pieces of information. First, I told them that their doctor recommends they get the vaccine. Second, I emphasized that this was a new vaccine and that their doctor knew nothing more about the vaccine than they, the patients, did. Despite this previous piece of information, people couldn't shake the suspicion that their doctor knew something that they didn't. I told them that the choice depended only on their own values. I re-emphasized that their doctor didn't know anything more about the vaccine than we were reporting here. And they still chose to get the vaccine if their doctor recommended it.

The power of recommendations is quite real, and not merely an artifact of experimental surveys. Consider the framing effect I discussed earlier that causes people to look more favorably on a surgical procedure with a 90 percent survival rate than on one with a 10 percent mortality rate. Laura Siminoff, a medical communications expert, led a research group that set out to determine how often such framing effects influence breast cancer patients deciding whether to take chemotherapy to reduce the chance of recurrence. Siminoff figured that when physicians framed outcomes negatively ("The cancer has a 15 percent chance of recurring"), women would choose more aggressive forms of adjuvant therapy than when physicians framed them positively ("There is an 85 percent chance you will be cured of the cancer").

But the framing effect—one of the most robust findings in the field of decision psychology and behavioral economics—was nowhere to be seen. No matter how doctors framed their options, whether positively or negatively, the frame didn't influence women's decisions. Instead, it was the doctor's recommendation that ruled the day.

Now, there are recommendations and there are *recommendations*. One doctor might gently recommend a treatment ("I think tamoxifen is the way to go, but I understand if you don't want to take an extra pill every day"), while another sternly offers advice ("You should take tamoxifen. That is what I recommend"). And there are morally important differences between these styles. Demeanor matters. Dogmatic-sounding pronouncements, even when couched as recommendations, don't differ from old-fashioned paternalism. Style is substance in doctor–patient interaction.

But even a gentle recommendation can have a very strong influence on a patient's choice. Patients read a lot into doctors' advice. Even when the right choice depends on more than medical facts—depends, in fact, on patient preferences—many patients mistakenly assume that physician recommendations are objective scientific pronouncements pointing them toward incontrovertible medical facts. Often this assumption is far from the truth.

WHAT YOU SEE IS WHAT YOU KNOW

With our recorder running on the desk between him and the patient, the urologist explained that the patient's tumor was slow-growing and treatable. He said that radiation would kill the prostate cancer cells without any need for a surgical incision. And then he shifted his attention to the next treatment. "Well, that's radiation, and of course if you want to learn more about radiation treatment, we can set up an appointment at the radiation clinic. But now I want to tell you about surgery. I know more about surgery than radiation because I'm a surgeon, and as a surgeon I have to admit to being biased toward surgery. Anyway, with surgery, we make an incision about this long . . ."

What would you do if your surgeon admitted he was biased in favor of surgery?

It's impossible to judge the appropriateness of physician recommendations without taking on the issue of bias. Most often, when people fret about physician bias, they focus on the troublesome financial conflicts of interest that have tainted the profession. These conflicts of interest are woven into the very fabric of medical practice in the United States, where doctors are paid on a fee-for-service basis: do more procedures and make more money. When U.S. surgeons say, "I think you need a prostatectomy," savvy patients are left to wonder whether the recommendation is being influenced, consciously or unconsciously, by the surgeon's desire to pay their children's college tuition. Most experts believe, in fact, that U.S. health costs consistently outpace inflation in no small part because of our crazy reimbursement system, which encourages doctors to do too many tests and procedures.

Even more concerning is that many physicians around the globe have entered into shadier financial relationships with drug companies and device manufacturers, relationships that give them incentives to recommend expensive drugs and devices to their patients. The *New York Times* documented one such relationship in the summer of 2011, describing how a company called Biotronik hired cardiologists to conduct what were essentially useless clinical trials so that the cardiologists would be more likely to recommend their pacemakers to patients. Even cardiologists who weren't in the pacemaker business came under the spell of Biotronik's influence. One general cardiologist received a couple thousand dollars a month from Biotronik and made it known to his pacemaker-implanting colleagues that he wouldn't refer his patients to them unless they promised to use Biotronik devices. It's hard to have faith in physician recommendations when doctors are focused so much on the bottom line.

But physician bias is much more insidious than these financial temptations. The urologist I quoted above, who admitted to being biased in favor of surgery over radiation, was a salaried employee of the VA health system. Adding another operation to his workload wouldn't give him a cent of additional money. And as a VA employee, his financial relationships with for-profit health-care companies were closely monitored. Therefore, when he said he was biased in favor of surgery, he wasn't admitting to a nefarious financial conflict of interest. He was just acknowledging that he liked what he knew and that he knew more about surgery than radiation. In fact, surveys have shown that urologists typically believe that surgery is the best treatment for localized prostate cancer, whereas radiation oncologists believe that radiation treatment is the best option.

This know-what-you-see bias probably explains why an orthopedic surgeon once told me that physical therapy wouldn't help one of my injuries, a statement he backed up by noting all the patients he'd operated on who had failed to improve with such therapy. What he didn't note, and may not have considered at the time, is that patients who improve with physical therapy are less likely to schedule follow-up visits in his clinic. The patients he saw as an orthopedic surgeon were not representative of patients as a whole.

As a primary care physician, I am susceptible to this same bias. For example, I have cared for many oncology patients with tumors that have progressed despite aggressive anticancer treatments, leaving me to coordinate their end-of-life care. Because of those experiences, I hold a less positive view of cancer therapy than a typical oncologist, who cares for many patients in outpatient chemotherapy centers, patients who never require hospitalization under the likes of me.

Not only do doctors know what they see but also, when informing patients about treatment options, they typically discuss what they know. The urologists I've tape-recorded often spend twice as much time discussing surgery as radiation. Compounding this imbalance in discussion time is an imbalance in positive and negative information, with physicians usually spending substantially more time laying out the benefits of their treatments than the risks.

Where does this leave patients? Seeking guidance from professionals whose knowledge of the decision at hand far exceeds their own, patients unwittingly find themselves on the receiving end of opinions potentially biased by financial interest or even by the whims of professional experience. Based on the problems inherent in physician recommendations, a patient would be justified in dismissing such recommendations altogether—not because all doctorly advice is necessarily and universally biased, but because an individual patient has no way of knowing which advice to trust. Yet given the potential benefits we've seen in getting advice from doctors, patients might want to consider a less extreme response to these problems. For starters, they can look to see whether their physician understands them well enough to give advice that fits their needs and desires. Because, as it turns out, physicians don't always understand their patients well enough to provide helpful recommendations.

KNOW YOUR AUDIENCE

Thomas Pohler sat in near silence for most of the visit, like so many of the other patients who have participated in our research. He didn't say much after the urologist told him he had prostate cancer. He didn't say much more when the oncologist explained the pros and cons of his treatment options. And now it was time to make a decision, or at least give the urologist a sense of his leanings, but Pohler couldn't make up his mind. So he asked the urologist for advice.

"What, in your opinion . . . which do you think would be best?"

The urologist refused to take the bait. "So, what we usually tell people is it's a decision that you've got to make."

"Right," Pohler responded, not sounding too gleeful about the thought of becoming an empowered decision maker.

The urologist, perhaps sensing his hesitancy, quickly continued. "But—and this is pretty much my bias because I am a surgeon—we tend to steer people who are older and sicker toward radiation as they are not going to recover from surgery well."

"Right," said Pohler, sounding relieved.

"Younger, healthier guys—guys like you—are people that are good candidates for the surgery . . . so, looking at you, I would tend to steer you toward surgery." The urologist's medical opinion, based on clinical facts, had led him to recommend surgery. Yet he still felt uncomfortable being so prescriptive: "But again, like I said, this is a decision that *you* have to make." Then the urologist asked a seemingly innocent question. "And now, how bad is your lung disease?"

"My what?"

"On your chart here, I notice that you have some lung disease? It says you have COPD [a medical acronym for emphysema]."

The surgeon had recommended surgery to Mr. Pohler—a recommendation based in large part on Pohler's healthiness and youth, a medically based recommendation—even though the surgeon didn't know whether Pohler had emphysema, the kind of serious lung disease that could make surgery a much riskier option. Good advice depends on good understanding. An advice giver who doesn't understand his advisee is in no position to provide wise counsel.

What is stunning to me about this conversation is that the urologist provided his patient with a treatment recommendation before understanding the medical facts of the case. Even in the old days of physician paternalism I wouldn't have expected that. In those times, you'll remember, doctors mistakenly believed that medical decisions were purely *medical* decisions, with the right choice depending solely on clinical facts. Prompted by that belief, they felt obligated to sort out these facts before telling patients what treatments they should receive. In the new paradigm, doctors have been taught that the right choice depends not only on clinical facts but also on patient preferences. Yet in this encounter the urologist not only failed to sort out the clinical facts before chiming in with his recommendation, he also delivered the recommendation without first eliciting Pohler's preferences. He didn't ask Pohler how bothered he would be by experiencing impotence or incontinence, or how worried he would be about leaving the cancer untreated for the while to see if it progresses. Having not assessed his patient's cares and worries, how can the urologist make a worthwhile recommendation?

Sometimes physicians fail to assess patient preferences because they are convinced that they know what patients want. Consider a study of conversations between gynecologists and their patients led by Sue Fisher from Wesleyan University. Fisher was studying patients who had abnormal pap smears, a finding that usually signifies that the patients have precancerous lesions on their cervix. Women have many options for what to do in response to an abnormal pap smear, options that vary in aggressiveness and in side-effect rates such that the best choice often depends on (you know this by now!) an individual patient's preferences. But Fisher did not come across many examples of gynecologists patiently questioning their patients about their preferences. Instead, most of the gynecologists assumed that they could deduce patients' preferences from the facts at hand. For example, the gynecologists routinely asked women how many children they had. From this information they made unjustified leaps of logic. If a woman said she had several children already, the doctor would recommend a hysterectomy, believing that the desire to have more children would be outweighed, in these women, by the chance to rid themselves of any cancer. If a woman hadn't had babies yet, she'd receive a less aggressive treatment so that she would not lose the chance of becoming pregnant. In most of the encounters, the gynecologists didn't try to find out how each patient felt about the treatment options before making treatment recommendations.

This lack of understanding caught up with one of the doctors when her patient came in for a pre-op visit and expressed second thoughts about her impending hysterectomy. "I'm terrified of operations," the woman said. The gynecologist was surprised but quickly recovered. "Uh, okay, well . . . there certainly *is* an alternative, yeah. We can treat this by just freezing it here in the office, and that usually will take care of it about 90 percent of the time."

The patient gladly opted for this less invasive treatment, a procedure she would not have learned about had she failed to express her concerns so explicitly. Unfortunately, most of the patients in Fisher's study were not so assertive.

THE KEY TO GOOD ADVICE

Good medical decision making requires good communication, and good communication flows in two directions. It's not enough for physicians to communicate clinical information to patients in a comprehensible manner; they also need to understand their patients' perspectives. Later, I'll discuss what it will take to change doctors' attitudes so that more of them strive for such understanding. But patients also need to change their mind-set. A patient cannot be content to absorb and comprehend what the doctor has told him about his medical condition. He also needs to make sure the doctor understands his point of view, his take on the relative pros and cons of the treatment alternatives. Would you take advice from a financial planner who hadn't taken the time to find out at what age you were planning to retire? Or from one who hadn't spoken with you about your willingness to pursue risky investments? Then don't take advice from a physician who has not taken the time to understand what you care about. Patients won't get good advice from their doctors if they don't find a way to make their preferences part of the conversation.

And how should patients go about doing this? They need to start by getting informed about their alternatives and, more specifically, about the role their preferences should play in the decision at hand. They need the power that comes with knowledge.

NINE

Empowering Patients with Information

It couldn't have been an easy video for Mary Smith to watch. It had been given to her by the staff at the Dartmouth-Hitchcock Medical Center because she'd been diagnosed with localized breast cancer and had an important decision to make. As explained in the video, initial treatment for early-stage breast cancer is surgical in nature. It involves removing the tumor by one of two methods, a mastectomy or a lumpectomy. A lumpectomy has the advantage of being a less invasive procedure. With a lumpectomy, the surgeon would leave most of her breast untouched and only remove the tumor (the lump that is being ectomied!). But lumpectomy carries a couple of disadvantages. Patients who receive lumpectomies typically need to undergo six weeks of radiation, traveling back and forth to the clinic each day for one hour of treatment, a treatment that can inflame a woman's skin and cause scar tissue to develop in the remainder of her breast. In addition, Smith would face a slightly increased chance of experiencing breast cancer recurrence. Not a pleasant thought to live with.

The biggest advantage of mastectomy is that it reduces the risk of recurrence while avoiding the need for radiation treatment. But choosing a mastectomy would mean saying good-bye to her breast forever.

If the video was difficult for Smith to watch, it was not because it was poorly produced. The video was a paragon of clarity and accessibility. Rather, the video was difficult to watch because it forced Smith to contemplate the harsh realities of her breast cancer. Watching someone describe a mastectomy, even when the description is elegant in its simplicity, is not easy to do when you realize it's *your* body that will soon end up on the operating-room table, *your* breast that may soon be removed from your body. Adding to the emotions caused by the video would have probably been another difficult feeling: the realization that she had to make a tough decision involving the kinds of trade-offs she had never had to confront before. Mastectomy or lumpectomy . . . which would it be?

It's no wonder that many patients in Smith's situation see the choice between mastectomy and lumpectomy as a lose-lose proposition. Nevertheless, Smith's situation required a choice and, having now watched the video and having spoken with her surgical oncologist, she made up her mind. She decided on a mastectomy.

Then Smith met with E. Dale Collins Vidal, a plastic surgeon at Dartmouth and, by coincidence, one of the people who had helped pilot-test the breast cancer video when it was first produced. Smith's decision didn't sit well with Collins Vidal because it didn't jibe with what she understood about Smith's preferences. You see, shortly after watching the video, Smith filled out a questionnaire assessing her attitudes toward the pros and cons of her treatment alternatives. Collins Vidal had taken care of many patients with breast cancer, and she had discovered that their answers to these questions typically lined up with the treatment they ended up having. Women who said they were anxious about breast cancer recurrence, for example, tended to choose mastectomy. Collins Vidal noticed that Smith's choice didn't match her survey responses. So she asked her to look over the video a second time, to make sure she was happy with her choice.

When they spoke again several days later, Smith had changed her mind. She told Collins Vidal that she had initially chosen mastectomy because that's what her surgical oncologist had recommended. But after watching the video again and thinking about her own prefer-ences, she realized that she wanted a lumpectomy. It was her choice, after all, not the surgeon's.

In the old days, Smith would have received the mastectomy her surgical oncologist had recommended. But Smith avoided that fate for two reasons. First, she encountered an enlightened physician in Collins Vidal, who embraced the idea of shared decision making. I'll return to the importance of such enlightened physicians in a later chapter. But for now, I'm going to focus on the second reason Smith was able to avoid an unnecessary mastectomy: She was given the opportunity to view a video program—an interactive decision aid—designed to empower her to participate in this decision.

Mary Smith was diagnosed with breast cancer in 2008, a time by which several hundred thousand patients in the United States had al-ready made use of decision aids to contemplate everything from rela-tively mundane decisions, such as whether to take a cholesterol pill, to more dramatic decisions, such as which breast cancer treatment to choose. The number of patients using decision aids has grown steadily over the years, both in the United States and across much of Europe. Decision aids have become a central part of efforts to promote shared decision making.

But despite this steady growth in use, the vast majority of patients facing important medical decisions will make those choices, or accede to the wishes of their physicians, without the benefit of a decision aid. According to the National Cancer Institute, over 200,000 women are diagnosed with invasive breast cancer annually in the United States alone. Add to that the 150,000 people diagnosed with colon cancer, the 200,000-plus diagnosed with lung cancer, and the almost 250,000 di-agnosed with prostate cancer and we're beginning to approach one mil-lion people in the United States alone who could benefit from the use of a decision aid to sort through their cancer treatments. Now, consider all the other health problems that confront patients with difficult decisions, from whether to take cholesterol pills to deciding whether to have a hip replacement. In most years, millions of adults in the United States and elsewhere could potentially benefit from decision aids. Yet only several hundred thousand patients have ever made use of decision aids. The fact is decision aids are still uncommon in medical practice. Most doctors haven't incorporated them into their daily routines and most patients haven't heard of them.

Smith had access to a decision aid because she received her care at Dartmouth University, home to an iconoclastic physician—Jack Wennberg—who gave birth to the idea of decision aids. What compelled Wennberg to create decision aids? It wasn't his experience with breast cancer patients per se, or those with high cholesterol. Nor was it any training he received in bioethics or health-care law. Instead, it all began with what started off as an innocuous study of hospital data in Vermont.

SMALL TOWNS WITH BIG DIFFERENCES

Wennberg was born in Bellows Falls, Vermont, just as the United States was coming out of the Great Depression. The son of a paper mill manager, he spent his youth skiing, snowshoeing, and reading Ibsen, almost as if he were growing up in his father's home country of Norway. A brilliant child, he excelled in school, graduating near the top of his medical school class and enrolling in residency in the early 1960s at Johns Hopkins University, one of the most prestigious medical centers in the world.

While at Johns Hopkins he provided an early demonstration of his willingness to challenge medical authority. He was taking care of a patient with unexplained kidney failure, and rather than treat the patient's illness and head home for the day, he found himself wondering what could have caused this man's illness. He obtained all the usual blood tests and X-rays, but no answer was forthcoming, which left Wennberg concerned that the patient's kidneys had been harmed by a new medication. Studies up to that time hadn't proven any connection between that medicine and kidney problems, but Wennberg wasn't satisfied. So, in the little spare time available to him as a medical resident, he began injecting cats with the drug to see what would happen—five milligrams in one cat, ten milligrams in another. When the cats began dying of kidney failure, he knew he'd found the culprit. Wennberg quickly sought out leaders at Johns Hopkins and pleaded with them to alert the FDA to the potential dangers of this drug. But no one at Johns Hopkins felt compelled to contact the authorities.

Undeterred, he wrote a letter to the manufacturer of the drug. When the manufacturer didn't reply, he wrote directly to the FDA, urging the agency to pull the drug from the market. His exhortations were met with deafening silence, but once again Wennberg was not ready to give up. He knew that something had to be done to prevent this medication from harming other patients.

So he wrote to Senator Hubert Humphrey, the famously energetic Minnesota liberal who would soon become vice president of the United States. Something in the letter must have hit home with Humphrey, because the senator took Wennberg's note to the White House, beginning a cascade of activity that ended only when the company voluntarily withdrew the drug from the market. Wennberg's persistence had paid off. Hundreds, perhaps thousands of people had been spared kidney failure because the young doctor wouldn't back down.

Persistence is a trait that has characterized Wennberg throughout his adult life, a trait he needed in large supply when he started uncovering previously unknown truths about how doctors made decisions about treatments like tonsillectomies. Imagine for a moment that a four-year-old, let's call him Johnny Tonsils, is suffering from a sore throat, his fourth such infection in the previous six months.

Johnny's neck is swollen from enlarged glands (lymph nodes, in medical vernacular), and his throat is red and raw from inflammation.

The doctor peers inside his mouth and catches sight of his swollen tonsils, which look really peeved at their current situation.

It is decision time. Should the doctor continue treating each of Johnny's infections with antibiotics or send him to a surgeon for a tonsillectomy? The medical facts alone don't point to a best choice. Surgery carries real pros and cons. It would eliminate future episodes of tonsillitis, but Johnny might still come down with other throat and ear infections. Plus, the surgery carries risks of pain, wound infection, and on rare occasions even more serious complications. And Johnny is nearing an age when many children stop having so many infections; their immune systems are finally robust enough to handle all those daycare germs.

Ideally, the physician would discuss the pros and cons of a tonsillectomy with Johnny's parents and decide together what would be in his best interests. Yet Jack Wennberg had developed a troubling suspicion that decisions about medical interventions, like tonsillectomies, weren't being made this way. It was the late 1960s, and Wennberg had returned to Vermont to become a director of that state's regional medical program, which had been created as part of Lyndon Johnson's Great Society with the goal of making sure everyone in the United States had access to the newest and greatest medical advances. At that time, Vermont's population numbered less than half a million people. It was a mostly rural state of dairy farmers and miners (and Ibsen enthusiasts, of course). Most acute medical care in Vermont took place in one of its community hospitals, meaning that when a Vermonter came down with a touch of pneumonia or a bout of rheumatoid arthritis, she would be admitted to the closest hospital, the same hospital she'd go to for a tonsillectomy or a hysterectomy. Despite being small and not very wealthy institutions, these hospitals had already developed advanced medical data systems due to the earlier leadership of a medical researcher at the University of Vermont. This data system was exactly what Wennberg used to uncover the strange ways in which doctors were making decisions about how to treat all of those little kids with sore throats.

Teaming up with Alan Gittelsohn, a statistician from Johns Hopkins, Wennberg began analyzing which patients were receiving which treatments at which hospitals. He set out to see if rural Vermonters had reduced access to new medical technologies. Instead, he discovered something truly stunning. Despite the homogeneity of his state, which was almost completely made up of rural Caucasians, there were dramatic variations in the rate at which residents were receiving medical treatments. In one region of Vermont, for example, physicians performed 20 hysterectomies for every 10,000 women. In another area they performed three times as many. In one region 7 percent of kids had had their tonsils removed, while in another 70 percent had undergone a tonsillectomy—almost as if the only indication for a tonsillectomy was the existence of tonsils. (No Tonsils Left Behind?) A whole host of medical procedures were being performed across Vermont with unexplained geographical variation. Surgeons busily removed gallbladders in one corner of the state, while in other corners they could barely be bothered to concern themselves with this tiny organ.

Wennberg wondered what could be occurring to justify such different rates of medical intervention. Were patients sicker in some areas of the state than others? Wennberg didn't think so. He didn't know of any epidemic of strep infections, for example, that had created a need for urgent tonsillectomies in one region and not in others. Besides, absolutely nothing he could think of could explain the threefold difference in hysterectomy rates across these regions. Fibroids and uterine cancer weren't contagious, after all. He was suspicious that the variation was caused by the way doctors made decisions.

A TALE OF TWO CONCUSSIONS

The ball thumped authoritatively off his right foot, and Jordan took off at full speed, hoping to turn his kick into an extra base hit. It was December in Michigan, but that didn't stop the fifth graders from playing kickball at recess. Jordan raced around first base and was ready to round second when—*phwoop!* He slipped on some ice. Black ice, as it turns out, a form of ice so dangerous even SEAL Team 6 trembles in its presence. His feet flew out from under him faster than even his young reflexes could respond, causing his head to slam onto the playground concrete with a dreadful-sounding *thwack*. The playground supervisor quickly rushed to his side and escorted the dazed ten-year-old to the school nurse's office.

I arrived twenty minutes later, having received a call from the nurse explaining that my son Jordan was acting strangely. By the time I arrived, Jordan had lost all memory of the accident. He had the classic signs of a concussion—headache, poor concentration, and absolutely no short-term memory. He didn't even remember the Michigan–Duke basketball game from the preceding week, a game at which he'd joined others in storming the court after Michigan's surprise victory.

"How did I hurt my head, Dad?"

"Playing kickball, Jordan."

"Oh, I see. Is that why we're in the nurse's office?" Fifteen seconds of unrelated conversation followed, then, "How did I hit my head, Dad?"

"Playing kickball, Jordan."

"Oh, I see. Is that why . . ."

The conversation continued cycling in this manner while I gathered his personal belongings and told his homeroom teacher I was taking him to the hospital's emergency room. (I was levelheaded enough to recognize that only a fool has his son for a patient.)

The emergency physician who examined Jordan reassured me that his concussion wasn't severe. Before sending him home, however, he wanted to make sure that the fall hadn't triggered any intracranial bleeding. So he whisked Jordan over to the CT machine, where his confidence in Jordan's prognosis was affirmed. No bleeding. Time to go home, but no roughhousing for a while.

Four weeks later, Jordan was back up to his roughhousing ways, wrestling with his third-grade brother, Taylor, in our living room while I played piano. (Nothing like Beethoven to rile up the boys.) Things were getting hectic, even by their standards, so I stopped playing piano and asked them to quiet down. Not heeding my direction, Taylor took one last charge at his big brother, a huge joy-of-the-battle grin spreading across his face as he leapt toward his opponent. Jordan is nothing if not a determined warrior, and he deflected his little brother's advance with a push that sent Taylor crashing backward, hitting his head so hard I could hear the floorboard rattle under two layers of carpeting. Taylor started crying, and I rushed to his side in full-paranoia mode, given Jordan's recent concussion. I tested his vision and his hearing. I asked him some questions and he answered coherently. So I told him to take it easy for a while, and he headed up to his bedroom to read.

Thirty minutes later, Jordan sought me out to tell me that Taylor was driving him crazy. "Dad, will you tell Taylor to stop asking me the same questions over and over again?" I had a second concussion on my hands.

I drove Taylor to the emergency room, where he demonstrated symptoms identical to his brother's four weeks earlier. Mild headache? Check. Loss of memory? Yep. Poor attention span? Three for three. Just like Jordan, Taylor had experienced a mild concussion, with no other signs or symptoms—no nausea, vomiting, or dizziness—to cause concern. The emergency physician explained that Taylor would recover on his own without any further treatment. In addition, he assured me that there was no need for further testing. "A CT scan," he told me, "would only expose him to potentially harmful radiation."

Huh? I had gone twice to the same emergency room, toting along children with identical signs and symptoms, and the doctors had made completely different recommendations about the necessity—or lack thereof—of an expensive and harmful CT scan. Almost forty years after Jack Wennberg's Vermont study, his research on variation in medical procedures was staring me in the face.

BLAMING PATIENTS

When Jack Wennberg discovered regional variations in medical care across the state of Vermont, no medical journal would publish his findings, because reviewers and editors were all convinced that there was a logical, medical explanation for these variations. They couldn't shake the suspicion that differences in age or race or illness or . . . *something* had led patients in some regions to need or demand more medical care than those in other regions. In 2008, when my boys experienced those two concussions, I had witnessed that different doctors make different decisions, despite identical medical circumstances. But Wennberg couldn't publish his findings because no one believed that doctors were responsible for the variations he had found.

Wennberg once again drew upon his seemingly inexhaustible reserve of persistence. A reviewer would criticize some aspect of his statistical analysis and, rather than give up, Wennberg would conduct further analyses to test for alternative explanations. A journal editor would suggest that his paper was not worth publishing because he had forgotten to look at such and such, and Wennberg would promptly pore over his files, looking for that supposedly overlooked such and such, find that it didn't explain his results, and resubmit the article to the journal. Inevitably, the editor would discover some new so-called flaw in Wennberg's revised article: "Sorry. Not up to the standards of *JAMA* (*Journal of the American Medical Association*)," *NEJM* (*New England Journal of Medicine*), etc. No statistical test would shake the establishment's belief that the variations in medical care Wennberg had identified were a result of variations in illness.

Wennberg harbored his own very different suspicions. He believed that the same health conditions were being treated differently by different doctors, just as the two emergency room physicians had cared differently for my two concussed boys. He believed that doctors didn't have consistent thresholds for when to perform specific medical procedures. Some surgeons might remove a patient's gallbladder when there was just the slightest concern that it was inflamed while other surgeons, presented with similar patients, held off on the operation. In short, Wennberg wasn't prepared to blame regional variations on patients—their illnesses or their demands. He thought the explanation lay inside physicians' brains.

Wennberg's beliefs did not make him popular among his colleagues. He'd present his research at medical conferences, explaining that he couldn't find any clinical explanation for his findings, and the audience would invariably pounce. Their defensiveness was understandable. After all, he was effectively accusing them of making arbitrary, even unscientific decisions about how to treat their patients. Wennberg's bosses weren't too happy with his findings either. In their eyes, his research was making the whole state of Vermont look bad. So they cut his research funding and moved him to a smaller office. When that didn't shut him up, they moved him to an even smaller office. Meanwhile, the poor guy still couldn't find a medical journal willing to publish his article.

In 1973, Wennberg decided to try his luck at a nonmedical journal and finally found an editor willing to publish his research. That journal was *Science,* arguably the most prestigious scientific journal in the world. His paper is now one of the most highly cited papers in the history of health policy.

But Wennberg wasn't content to publish this lone paper. His cranium was still stuffed with all those reviewer criticisms, telling him that the variations he'd found were the result of "patient factors." And even though none of his analyses confirmed the reviewers' beliefs, he knew that the data he had available to him couldn't eliminate the possibility that patient factors were behind the results. It was time to collect more data.

By the time *Science* published his first paper, Wennberg had moved from Vermont to Dartmouth, and while living in New Hampshire, he took the opportunity to make regular trips to Boston to collaborate with researchers in that medical metropolis. On one of those trips, he arranged to meet with Jack Fowler, a survey expert at the University of Massachusetts. Fowler was mesmerized by Wennberg, who spoke with such conviction about his discoveries that Fowler had no choice but to work with him. Together, they surveyed patients to find out whether differences in their health or in their desire for medical interventions would explain variations in the intensity of medical care they received.

Wennberg and Fowler's findings proved the critics wrong. Wherever they looked, the populations they surveyed looked the same. Not all patients were identical to each other, of course—some patients were relatively healthy while others were relatively sick; some were more inclined to seek medical care while others tried to avoid doctors at all costs—but these differences did not vary by geography. Where Wennberg had found threefold and fivefold differences in the receipt of medical procedures, he didn't find comparable differences in population needs or desires. The conclusion was inescapable: Women were receiving hysterectomies (and children were undergoing tonsillectomies) not because they were in need of such procedures, or even because they wanted such procedures, but because they happened to live in areas where doctors were in the habit of performing such procedures.

To understand what was so surprising about Wennberg's research, we must remember that in the early 1970s when he began this work, no one would have been shocked to learn that most medical decisions were being made by physicians. It was still the time of "doctor knows best." So when all those journals attributed Wennberg's findings to patient preferences, they were being disingenuous at best. They had to know that it wasn't the patients who were pushing doctors to make these strange decisions.

What was surprising about Wennberg's research, then, was not that doctors were making these decisions without regard to patient preferences but that doctors' decisions had so little to do with the medical facts of an individual patient's circumstances. It wasn't surprising that a woman's "decision" to get a hysterectomy was determined primarily by whether her doctor recommended such a procedure. But it was shocking to learn that it wasn't the "facts on the ground" that were determining these recommendations. It was the ground!

As Wennberg expanded his research from Vermont to all of the northeastern states, and from there to the entire country, the existence of regional variations would become indisputable, and the role of physician attitudes in driving such variations would become increasingly difficult to deny. In one study, for instance, Wennberg discovered a number of locations in the United States where women with early-stage breast cancer received a lumpectomy and a mastectomy in nearly equal proportions, while in other locations 98 percent of women received a mastectomy. A reporter followed up on this astonishing finding by interviewing surgeons in Rapid City, South Dakota, one of the locations where mastectomies ruled. She encountered a community of surgeons who were confident that they knew what was best for their patients. "As far as I'm concerned," one told her, "the gold standard is still mastectomy." Probably much the same attitude Mary Smith encountered many years later, when her surgical oncologist recommended she receive a mastectomy. But Smith ultimately rejected that advice, in part because she reviewed the breast cancer decision aid.

How, then, did Wennberg move from studying hospital data sets to promoting decision aids? That particular part of the story began during an evening stroll on Santa Monica beach.

OCEANSIDE DEBATE

The headquarters of the RAND Corporation stands just a few short blocks away from the Pacific Ocean, placing RAND about as far away from the center of U.S. politics as it is possible to be in the lower forty-eight states. Yet RAND has long been one of the most influen-

tial think tanks in the country, exerting an influence on U.S. policy
that belies both its location and its relatively modest size.

RAND is best known to most people for its work on military
strategy. The idea of MAD (mutually assured destruction)—whereby
the United States could prevent a Soviet nuclear attack by having the
means to destroy the former USSR in a counterattack—was developed
in large part by RAND thinkers. But those of us in medicine know
RAND best for its enormously influential health policy research. If a
research topic is relevant to health policy, you can bet that someone at
RAND has done seminal work in the area.

No doubt RAND researchers paid close attention to Jack Wennberg as he followed up his Vermont findings with studies exploring
variations across the United States, studies revealing that whole met-
ropolitan areas, whole regions of the country, had developed their own
practice styles. According to Wennberg's research, a person's chance of
receiving surgery for heart disease or back pain, or of receiving pills
for blood pressure or sore throats, depended as much on where they
lived—Miami or Cleveland; the Northeast versus the Southwest—as
it did on their medical histories. Over time, mainstream medical
journals began publishing Wennberg's studies. With each publica-
tion, Wennberg and his colleagues ramped up the sophistication of
their analyses until few experts could argue anymore that these variations were simply a matter of unmeasured illness or of variations in
patient preference.

Ultimately, the folks at RAND were so convinced of the validity
of Wennberg's research that they felt it was time to figure out what
could be done to reduce these unnecessary variations. In 1988, they
invited Wennberg and his colleagues to Santa Monica, hoping the two
groups could develop a joint solution to the problem.

Bob Brook, a monumental figure in health-care policy research, led
the RAND team. He'd played a crucial role in understanding what
happens when people lack health insurance. In addition, most modern

methods of measuring the quality of medical care—from the skill of your surgeon to the capability of your favorite community hospital—can be traced back to Brook's record. Brook made it clear, early in the meeting with Wennberg, that the key to reducing variations was to better educate doctors about what treatments were appropriate for given patients. He proposed to convene panels of physicians who would develop clinical practice guidelines describing, for example, when back pain should be treated by surgery versus physical therapy.

Wennberg, in contrast, didn't see how guidelines could solve the problem. Guidelines struck him as a modern way of taking decision-making power away from patients. He was worried that guidelines would medicalize decision making, a recipe for deciding on medical interventions that lacked a crucial ingredient: patient preferences. Since the right choice depends on what a given patient values, Wennberg argued, the *patient* needs to be at the center of any intervention.

The powwow turned out to be a disaster. The two great leaders—Brook and Wennberg—couldn't bridge the divide. Brook was adamant that the solution lay in physician guidelines; Wennberg insisted that patients needed to be at the center of any solution. Both men, known as much for their confidence as their brilliance, were too far apart to craft any kind of joint solution.

Frustrated by the stubbornness of the RAND team, Wennberg and his colleagues went for a walk on the beach. Jack Fowler joined Wennberg on that walk, as did Al Mulley, a physician at Harvard known for his clinical acumen, his research expertise, and his ability to turn a phrase. Wennberg was beside himself with the insolubility of the problem he had identified all those years ago in Vermont. "How can we change this?" he asked his friends. Mulley lobbied for putting information into patients' possession. He even had a slogan for such an approach: "Let the second opinion be your own." The problem, as Mulley saw it, was that the playing field wasn't level. Doctors had all the knowledge and thus all the power. Patients couldn't be expected to say no to unnecessary surgery until they were armed with the information that surgery was unnecessary.

BRINGING INFORMATION TO THE PEOPLE

When Wennberg and his colleagues walked on Santa Monica beach, they hatched the idea of decision aids. But ideas only change the world if people act upon them.

Act they did. Wennberg's team went right to work figuring out how to empower patients with knowledge. Soon they developed their first decision aid, an interactive computer videodisc designed to help men figure out whether to undergo surgery for benign prostatic hyperplasia (BPH)—a condition in which a man's prostate gland grows so large that it impairs his ability to urinate normally.

They chose BPH for several reasons. Wennberg's team had already learned that there were huge geographic variations in the rate of surgery for this condition. It was geographic variation that had spurred them on to create decision aids, so they naturally looked to these same variations to find clinical conditions in need of such an intervention. In addition, they had already conducted a decision analysis that had proved with what they viewed as mathematical certainty that the "right" choice in treating BPH often depended on patient preferences. Their goal in developing decision aids, after all, was to help patients make preference-sensitive choices. Finally, they had developed a good working relationship with a group of enlightened urologists who were willing to give the decision aid to their patients. Wennberg, Fowler, and Mulley were all idealists at heart, but idealists with strong pragmatic instincts. They knew they couldn't change the world without the help of a lot of other people.

With a topic in hand and a group of clinicians willing to collaborate, Wennberg's team now had to figure out what the decision aid should look like. They could simply print a detailed educational pamphlet, but that would risk alienating patients who weren't big readers. Plus, it would force the team to design a one-size-fits-all intervention, with every patient receiving the same information regardless of the specifics of their disease. Then they came up with the idea of an interactive videodisc. Remember, the Internet was not in widespread use in the late 1980s. People couldn't turn to websites for information or view a YouTube video. The interactive videodisc worked almost like a small website that people could download to their home computers. With the disc, Wennberg's team was able to individually tailor information to match each patient's needs. Patients would enter information about their age and their symptoms into their computer, or a computer made available to them at their local medical clinic, and the video program would spin to the section of the decision aid most relevant to their situation.

Now it was time to figure out what information to communicate in the decision aid. Their goal was not information for information's sake. Wennberg's team wanted to provide information to patients so they would be empowered. Consequently, they began the decision aid by emphasizing the centrality of each patient's values in determining the right choice: "There is a decision to be made by you and your doctor. How you decide depends on how you feel . . . about the possible harms and benefits of surgery compared to the possible harms and benefits of watchful waiting." Only after giving this empowerment pep **talk did** the decision aid begin informing patients about the treatment options, laying out the odds of various harms and benefits accompanied by colorful pie charts.

Recognizing that all this statistical mumbo jumbo could quickly become a snooze fest, they supplemented the narrative with testimonials from two patients who'd gone through this decision, one who had chosen surgery and the other who had chosen to wait. With these testimonials, they were able to give patients a better picture of what it feels like to make this decision and a more vivid idea of what it means to experience the harms and benefits of either treatment. For example, the patient who chose watchful waiting described how his decision to forgo surgery forced him to come up with methods of adapting to his symptoms. He explained one such method, a habit of ordering concert tickets "on the aisle side so I can get out in a hurry if I need to." The patient who chose surgery described some of the burdens of the procedure but also its benefits, including a compelling story about the way he greeted his urologist when returning to the clinic after his surgery. Delighted to be rid of his urinary symptoms, he broke into a Gershwin song. "Summertime," he sang, "and the peeing is easy."

The BPH decision aid was controversial. Many urologists were upset because patients who viewed the decision aid were less likely to undergo surgery. It was fine, in theory, to inform patients about their treatments, but the information in the decision aid was hurting their bottom line. The decision aid was received much more warmly by those outside the urology world. Many patient advocates were thrilled. It had been a decade and a half since the Karen Ann Quinlan case had dominated the news, and it felt to many enthusiasts like the patient-empowerment revolution had stalled. These newfangled decision aids struck many people as the key to completing the revolution.

In the years since the BPH videodisc, decision aids have proliferated dramatically. Moreover, research has shown that these decision aids have had a major impact on decision making. Decision aids consistently increase patient knowledge and often increase how satisfied patients are with their decisions. Sometimes decision aids change the decisions patients and their doctors make, with several trials demonstrating that patients who receive decision aids undergo less aggressive treatment than other patients.

That's not to say that decision aids have come even close to meeting their potential. As I discussed in the opening of this chapter, the vast majority of patients who could benefit from decision aids don't even know they exist. So far, there has been little money to be made designing and delivering decision aids. That's beginning to change, but there is still more money to be made by the U.S. health-care system when it performs unnecessary or unwanted procedures than when it provides patients with decision aids. In addition, there has been little political pressure to require that health-care providers give patients access to decision aids. Though that too is changing. Wennberg and his colleagues helped influence the state of Washington to mandate the use of decision aids in preference-sensitive decisions, a "soft" mandate that hasn't been fully implemented. They even convinced folks writing federal health-reform legislation in 2009 to include a couple of unfunded nods toward the importance of shared decision making.

It's tempting to think that patient empowerment is within our grasp, that with a few more laws or a bit more money decision aids will become the standard of care, thereby creating a world where informed and empowered patients exert their justly deserved influence on health-care decisions. But decision-aid advocates rarely talk about handing decisions over to empowered patients. Instead, they proselytize for the idea of shared decision making, with decision aids being used to improve the way doctors and patients talk about health-care alternatives. This emphasis on shared decision making isn't surprising given that three of those four men walking the Santa Monica beach that night were physicians. These doctors believed in empowering patients through information, but not in order to relegate physicians to the role of information clarifier. They recognized that physicians would almost always play a central role in medical decision making. They just wanted to make sure patients had enough information at their disposal to partner with their physicians, so that those patients' preferences would become part of the conversation.

I am a huge fan of decision aids. Nevertheless, I don't think that widespread use of these interventions, in their current form, will bring us where we need to be. To date, decision aids have largely been designed by people—brilliant, rational people, many of whom are ex-

perts in fields like decision analysis—who believe that information is
the key to shared decision making. But information does not necessarily lead to activation. Decision aids won't meet their full potential if
the only thing they accomplish is to increase patient knowledge. They
also need to change behavior. And to do that, they need to better account for the ways in which people make decisions once they've been
informed about their alternatives.

TEN

Aligning Information
with Behavior

Poor old Harry Hypothetical has a decision to make and he needs your help. Harry suffers from a severe case of acute hotchocolitis, a dreaded condition that he is desperate to be cured of. But there is no obvious "best" treatment for Harry. He has two legitimate options, each with its risks and benefits. He could take a medication called Chocoway or its competitor Hotnomore. Both pills would cure his disease, but at a risk of experiencing one of two side effects. Both medications can cause spasmodic spleen syndrome. (You don't want to know the details about this imaginary condition.) This side effect occurs in 20 percent of people taking Chocoway and 30 percent taking Hotnomore. Both pills also carry a risk of intermittent thyroidal retaliation syndrome, a side effect that occurs in 40 percent of Chocoway users versus only 20 percent of people taking Hotnomore.

The right choice for Harry clearly depends on how he views the relative undesirability of these two side effects, traded off against the likelihood that each pill would cause the side effects. To make that choice, Harry needs to understand what each of these side effects would feel like. At the same time he needs to comprehend the odds of experiencing either side effect should he choose one treatment over the other. That's where your help comes in. Harry needs you to design a decision aid that will help him make this choice. And that means you have a few decisions of your own to make.

Let's start with those side effect numbers. How do you want to present those statistics to Harry? Remember, like many people, Harry struggles to understand concepts like probability and percentages. He never excelled in high school math and he has a hard time balancing his checkbook. What words would you use to inform Harry that he faces a 20 percent chance of spasmodic spleen syndrome if he takes Chocoway? Would you complement those words with a picture? If so, what kind of picture? A pie chart? A bar graph? And which side effect would you describe first, the one more common with Chocoway or the one more common with Hotnomore? Will Harry quickly make up his mind before learning about the two side effects?

As we saw in part II, the feel of risk can be influenced by subtle changes in the way people receive information. A treatment with a 90 percent survival rate feels better than one with a 10 percent mortality rate. A pill that causes side effects in 320 out of 1,000 people feels riskier than one that causes side effects in 32 out of 100. You have a tough job ahead of you, to give Harry this information in a manner that won't bias his choice. But there is more. In addition to explaining the risks of these two side effects, you also need to explain what it will feel like to experience them. How will you help Harry imagine the impact that intermittent thyroidal retaliation will have on his life? Too many words and you will lose your audience, but too few words and you'll leave Harry in the dark. Or would you largely abandon words to describe either of these side effects and stick with video images—interviews, say, with people who've lived with these syndromes? Would it matter who you interviewed? Would it need to be someone of the same age and race and gender as Harry? Do you need a whole catalogue of interviewees so that every person who views your decision aid will have exposure to testimonials from someone to whom they can relate?

Lots of design decisions to make, each with the potential to influence Harry's choice. Rather daunting, isn't it? You set out with the noble goal of helping Harry pick the treatment that best fits his individual preferences, and now you have to worry that the way you describe his options—even the mere order in which you present information—could unduly influence his choice.

The decision-aid movement, as we have seen, has been led by people who believe in the power of information. And it's hard to quibble with the idea of helping patients understand their treatment alternatives. Better for someone like Harry to hear about the side effects of these two drugs, in one order or another, than to never learn about them at all. Nevertheless, decision aid design matters. It is now being influenced by behavioral scientists like me, people who are obsessed with irrational decisions and who want to design decision aids that reduce the chance that people will be biased by the information contained within. A quick tour of some de-biasing techniques will illustrate the power of behavioral science to work toward the goal of promoting shared decision making.

ANECDOTAL REASONING

I wasn't trying to be pushy, but I really thought that Mr. Floyd would benefit from a statin, a cholesterol pill that would significantly reduce his chance of experiencing a second heart attack. The pill wouldn't cost Mr. Floyd much money. And he'd only have to take it once a day. True, he'd probably have to take it for the rest of his life, and the pill might cause him to experience transient liver problems, but these problems typically resolve quickly with cessation of treatment. Floyd wasn't concerned about liver problems though. He was worried about muscle and kidney damage. His best friend had experienced an unusually bad response to a statin. His muscles had broken down in the presence of the drug, and proteins from the damaged tissue had circulated in the bloodstream until they had crammed themselves into his kidney tubules, causing irreversible damage to those critical organs.

I tried to reason with Mr. Floyd. "I'm really sorry to hear about your friend. He had really awful luck. I think what he experienced is really rare. I've given these pills to hundreds of patients, and I've never had one who experienced that big of a problem." Floyd was not persuaded. I explained that we could monitor him for early signs of such a side effect. "We can test for muscle enzymes in your blood. And if you feel any, *any* kind of muscle aches after taking the pill, you can stop taking it right away. We can then find a pill that won't cause such problems for you."

He was still not persuaded. "I don't like what that pill did to my friend, and I don't want it doing that to me." In other words: Not. Gonna. Happen.

No doubt every practicing clinician has experienced a version of this encounter. A patient reports the experience of a friend or relative who had an unusual response to a treatment, and this friend's experience makes it impossible for the clinician to convince the patient that their story won't have the same ending. The well-intentioned clinician tries to counter with hard data: "Only 1 percent of people have that reaction." But how can statistics compete with anecdotes?

The history of humankind is much more closely linked to stories than to numbers. For generations humans passed knowledge on through storytelling, long before the invention of the written word and still longer before the invention of mathematics and statistics. Stories remain central to human experience. The most talented journalists and politicians of today, perhaps recognizing this history, don't rely on numbers and figures to engage audiences. They tell stories.

In a classic example of the power of anecdotes, Richard Nisbett and Lee Ross, two giants in the field of social psychology, presented information to a group of students who were trying to decide what classes to take that semester. They gave students detailed data on how previous students had rated each available course. Then they asked a few previous students to tell anecdotes about what they thought of the courses. Nisbett and Ross discovered that these brief testimonials had a disproportionate impact on students' course choices. The data were too bland to compete with these in-person reviews.

Think about the importance of this phenomenon in the context of designing decision aids. Many decision aids contain testimonials from patients who have already faced the decision in question. The patients often describe their experiences—what it felt like to recover from surgery, for example, or to experience a treatment side effect. Decision aids typically go back and forth between these stories and treatment statistics—information about the probability of experiencing specific outcomes after choosing a given treatment. Can these outcome statistics compete with vivid stories?

To answer this question, I asked people to imagine that they had heart disease, which caused them to experience chest pain with exertion. I explained that there were two possible treatments for this condition, bypass surgery and balloon angioplasty. I described bypass surgery as an arduous procedure, requiring several days in the hospital and months of recovery. On the upside, I told them that it had a 75 percent chance of curing them of this illness. (The decision was strictly hypothetical, as were the outcome statistics that I asked them to contemplate.) I described the second treatment, balloon angioplasty, as being much less arduous, requiring an overnight stay in the hospital following the simple insertion of a catheter through their leg artery, a procedure they would recover from in one or two days. But I also told them it had only a 50 percent chance of curing their symptoms. A simple trade-off then: an arduous procedure with a 75 percent cure rate or an easier procedure with a 50 percent chance of cure. The best choice for any given person depends on how they feel about this trade-off. But my interest wasn't in their risk–benefit thinking per se. I wanted to see if that thinking would change if I told them some stories. After describing each treatment, I quoted several hypothetical patients who had undergone each procedure. The patients described whether the procedure had relieved them of their symptoms.

For instance, they might receive an anecdote from Bill H., age fifty-six: "I'd been having chest pains for about a year. It got so I couldn't even take a walk. Now that I've had my bypass, I'm walking to church again every Sunday. Praise the Lord!" They might receive one from Sally G., age sixty-one: "I'd always been active, until the angina stuff started. I hoped the bypass would cure me and get me out on the tennis courts again. But it didn't. Looks like game, set, and match for the angina."

I did all of the scientific stuff I needed to do to make sure that people weren't biased by the small details of the anecdote they received. Worrying that tennis players might react more to the tennis anecdote, I randomly varied whether or not the tennis player got better with the treatment across different versions of my survey. In other words, half the people making their hypothetical choice read about a tennis player who got better with treatment and the other half read about a tennis player who got no better with treatment. I also randomly varied whether the tennis player received the bypass surgery or the balloon angioplasty. I made the same kind of random variations for every other anecdote.

But there was one thing I didn't leave up to random chance. For each of the treatments, I included one story from a patient who benefitted and one from a patient who did not. Each participant read about one patient who had improved with a bypass, one who hadn't improved with a bypass, one who had improved with an angioplasty, and one who hadn't. After absorbing all of this information, only 20 percent of the people said they would opt for the bypass surgery and the remainder chose the angioplasty.

Was that the right choice? I can't judge that. Then again, my goal wasn't to see what people think about a bypass versus an angioplasty.

I wanted to see whether the anecdotes would unduly influence people's choices. In this particular case, I wondered whether the balance of anecdotes would overwhelm the actual statistical information. After all, the anecdotes made each treatment look like it worked 50 percent of the time, since one out of the two testimonials for each treatment came from someone with a happy ending. But the data explained that bypass surgery worked 75 percent of the time. I needed to figure out whether the mixture of happy and unhappy anecdotes was influencing people's choices.

So I ran an experiment. At the same time I gave some people the "balanced" mixture of fifty-fifty anecdotes, I gave another group statistically reinforcing anecdotes in which the success rate depicted in the anecdotes matched the statistics. For instance, I included four testimonials from people who had received bypass surgery, with three out of those four describing happy endings. And my experiment proved that the mix of anecdotes strongly influenced choice. The survey respondents who received these statistically reinforcing anecdotes were twice as likely to say they would choose bypass surgery.

What was striking about the study was that the anecdotes were completely uninformative. All the stories did was tell people whether or not a specific person got better with the treatment at hand. They already knew the actual percentage of people who would benefit from each treatment. In addition, when I described the treatments, I let them know that the angina might prevent them from activities such as walking to church or playing tennis. So the anecdotes provided *no additional information whatsoever.* Yet even the bland testimonials I used in my study—hardly as evocative as the kind of video interviews used in decision aids—still managed to overwhelm the statistical information. What can we do to make statistics more relevant to patients as they make important decisions?

A PICTURE IS WORTH A THOUSAND STATISTICS

Wennberg and his colleagues already had a notion when they designed the BPH decision aid that the statistical information they gave to patients wouldn't sink in unless they illustrated the statistics with images, like pie charts. Pie charts seemed like a logical choice at the time. They are uncluttered, especially when used to illustrate simple probabilities. Take information such as "Your chance of cure is 75 percent." That's quite easy to represent in a pie chart:

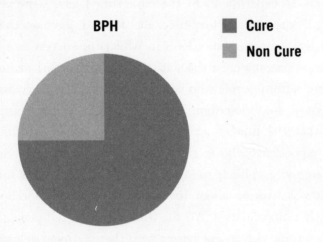

And people love pie charts, saying they are easy to use and understand. There is only one problem with people's love of pie charts. They leave many people confused. People who get information in the form of pie charts have a hard time giving accurate estimates of the risks being pictured. For example, my colleagues and I gave people information comparing the side-effect rates of two medications, illustrated with pie charts, and we discovered that many had a hard time telling us which pill was more likely to cause which side effect.

Fortunately, alternative graphical displays, like pictographs, are easy for people to understand and use. Pictographs help people get a feel for the specific numbers relevant to the decision. Consider the following pictograph:

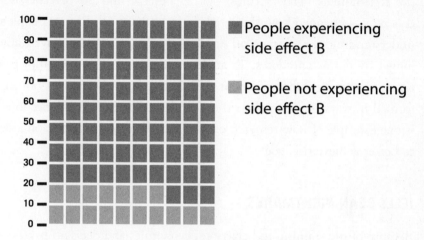

Most people who see this can very quickly tell you that 17 out of 100 people taking pill A experience side effect B. Better yet, the pictograph minimizes the chance of framing effects. If I tell you in words alone that 17 percent of people experience side effect B, you might not pay attention to the fact that 83 percent of people *won't* experience the side effect. But the pictograph reminds you about this 83 percent. That means the whole framing problem (a surgery with a 10 percent mortality rate is worse than one with a 90 percent survival rate) is minimized when people see pictographs displaying both survivors and nonsurvivors.

Behavioral scientists like me are working through the specifics about how best to inform patients about the risks and benefits of their treatment alternatives. If we want to involve patients in their decisions, then the devil is truly in the details of how we inform patients about their choices. In a study I ran with Angie Fagerlin we discovered that pictographs eliminate the anecdote problem. It no longer mattered whether the anecdotes reinforced the statistics. When we gave people pictographs, illustrating the 50 percent and 75 percent success rates of each treatment, the mix of anecdotes no longer influenced their choices. The pictograph was vivid enough to compete with the testimonials. The pictures—of 75 percent and 50 percent success rates—changed how these risks felt, perhaps solidifying people's understanding of the trade-off enough that they weren't swayed any longer by tennis anecdotes. To achieve true decision partnership, patients need to be informed about their health-care alternatives but informed in ways that don't bias their choices. My research on anecdotes is one example of how research can inform the design of decision aids to better achieve this goal.

JELLY BEAN NIGHTMARES

Because of my training in behavioral economics and decision psychology, my excitement at the arrival of Wennberg's decision aids had to compete with my fear and worry—fear that the design of the decision aids would bias people's choices and worry that these noble efforts to help patients make preference-sensitive decisions would instead unconsciously shape those same preferences. Take the graph shown on page 243. When I see that pictograph, itself already an improvement over Wennberg's pie charts, I don't just see 17 out of 100 boxes colored to represent some health outcome. I see jelly beans. I'm referring to the study I described in chapter 6 in which people hoping to pick a red jelly bean out of a jar had felt that the jar with 9 red jelly beans in a total of 100 was more alluring than the jar with 1 red one in a total of 10. I look at that pictograph and wonder: Will it inform choice or determine it?

Consider a group of patients taking a blood pressure pill over many years of time. Imagine that 16 percent of them experience stomach ulcers in the first five years of taking the pill. That sounds like a pretty high risk. But suppose I told you that 9 percent of those people would have experienced stomach ulcers over that same period of time even if they hadn't taken the medication. I know this is a lot of math, but bear with me for another minute, because you will someday face an important medical decision that requires you to wade through some math yourself. And I want to show you how behavioral scientists like me are trying to make that job easier.

The way decision aids would normally inform people about these stomach ulcers would be to tell you that 9 percent of people, at baseline, experienced these ulcers and that the medication increases that risk to 16 percent. The decision aid might even illustrate these two numbers with side-by-side pictographs, one showing 9 out of 100 boxes shaded in and the other showing 16.

As it turns out, when people view these side-by-side pictographs, they are highly susceptible to jelly-bean feelings. People who view a pictograph illustrating that 16 out of 100 people experience ulcers are less worried than people who view a pictograph illustrating that 160 out of 1,000 people will experience this same fate. For most people, 160 out of 1,000 is scarier than 16 out of 100.

These jelly-bean feelings are another challenge for patients facing important medical decisions, whose choices are being unduly influenced by arbitrary things like whether their risks are described as subsets of 100 or 1,000 (or some other denominator, for that matter). To make matters worse, it is not obvious which denominator is right. Perhaps when describing rare conditions it's useful to use a large denominator. But would such a denominator make sense for more common side effects, or would they make such side effects appear too scary? Finally, these side-by-side pictographs force people to figure out how many of those 16 (out of 100) ulcers are caused by the medication. The math is not difficult: 16 minus 9 equals 7. But many people I have shown this type of information to had a hard time doing the math. Moreover, even those who can figure out the math have to exert mental effort to do so, and this effort makes them more susceptible to jelly-bean logic.

Brian Zikmund-Fisher also found himself worrying about jelly-bean logic. Brian is one of my closest colleagues, a razor-sharp decision scientist who has dedicated his career to improving health-related decisions. Brian was a graduate student at Carnegie Mellon University in the late 1990s, studying economics and financial decision making, when he developed a rare and life-threatening bone marrow disorder. He had to put his graduate studies on hold in order to receive a bone marrow transplant, a bear of a treatment that he was lucky to survive. Brian faced a slew of decisions throughout his treatment course, and by the time he recovered from his illness, he had decided to use his scientific knowledge to help future patients make the decisions they would face.

Brian came to me one day with an idea about how to avoid the jelly-bean problem. The issue, as he saw it, was that side-by-side pictographs hide the math from people, thereby making them more susceptible to jelly-bean logic. Then he showed me an alternative. On a computer screen, he showed me a pictograph with the lower nine boxes shaded in dark blue, illustrating the pictograph I described earlier. As he hit the down arrow on the computer's keyboard, the next seven boxes changed in color from gray to light blue. The legend alongside the pictograph explained that the light blue boxes represented stomach ulcers caused by the medication. Brian's simple alteration of the pictograph had accomplished a potentially important goal—it had done the math for people.

Brian and I quickly went to work testing this new way of illustrating medication side effects. To one group of people, we presented the old side-by-side pictographs, the ones that didn't do the math for them. We found that jelly-bean logic ran rampant among this group of people. Those people who received pictographs with 100 squares in them were less worried than those whose pictographs had 1,000 squares, because the 16-out-of-100 risk felt less worrisome than the 160-out-of-1,000 risk.

But with another group of people, chosen at random from the population we surveyed, we made use of Brian's new pictograph, the one that used different colors to do the math for the viewer. In this group, jelly-bean reasoning was no longer evident. It no longer mattered whether we pictured risks as occurring out of 100 people or out of 1,000. Once again, we'd shown how a dose of behavioral science could minimize the impact of decision biases.

As decision aids mature, you can expect more of them to build on the insights of behavioral scientists. This means that when you get sick and have an important decision to make, you will have the chance to get informed about your choices without worrying that the decision-aid designer has unintentionally influenced your decision.

REIMAGINING THE UNIMAGINABLE

Brian Johnson is a lean, healthy-looking man in his early twenties. He stares into the camera and announces, matter-of-factly, that he is going to demonstrate what it is like to change a colostomy bag. Johnson (his real name, unlike most patients in this book) had lived with a severe case of Crohn's disease for many months, an inflammatory disease that had all but destroyed his colon. His illness was so advanced his doctors had needed to remove his entire colon and a good portion of his small intestine.

Johnson describes his life with an ostomy as rocky. "It started out being extremely difficult to deal with, but over time it has become second nature." In other words, he has largely adapted to his condition: "It is just a part of who I am now."

Part of the way Johnson coped with his illness was to turn outward, to focus on helping other people rather than turning inward to bemoan his own fate. He wanted other people with ostomies to "realize that they are not alone." That's what convinced Johnson to post a YouTube video in which he focused the camera on his belly while he removed his colostomy pouch, cleaned his skin (the pink protrusion of his stoma now visible to the world), and put on a replacement pouch. Johnson had made his video with the goal of helping people imagine what life would be like with a colostomy and to help new colostomy patients figure out how to more efficiently change their colostomy bags. (You can find this video at http://vimeo.com/36910721.)

A worthy goal. But would this video help or hinder people's ability to imagine life with a colostomy? Unknown to Johnson, Angelo Volandes, a medical researcher at Massachusetts General Hospital, had discovered that patient videos can do a tremendous job of improving people's ability to imagine otherwise unimaginable health conditions. During his clinical training, Volandes often felt himself frustrated when talking with patients about the kind of care they wanted to receive if they became too ill to participate in the decision. He would speak with people who had early signs of Alzheimer's disease, for example, and ask them whether, when they became too demented to communicate, they would want to be admitted to the hospital for aggressive treatment of acute illnesses. Many would confidently claim that they want "everything possible"—antibiotics, ventilators, even CPR. Volandes would inform them that, on a good day, people with end-stage Alzheimer's are unable to recognize their children, feed or clothe themselves, or even enjoy an episode of *Matlock* (God forbid!). Yet people would persist in wanting a full-court press. Volandes was convinced that people hadn't adequately imagined what life is like for people with severe dementia. So he decided to make a movie.

The video Volandes produced centers around an elderly woman who we physicians would describe as being "pleasantly demented." In contrast with many other people with dementia, she never appears agitated by her confusion. She stares ahead vacantly, unaware of her condition, oblivious to her environment. At one point in the video, her daughters are seated next to her, spooning lunch into her mouth as if she were an infant. She shows no signs of recognizing them, no clue that she has no clue. She is well dressed and well cared for, living in what looks like a good nursing home. In many ways, she is the best-case scenario for what life with end-stage Alzheimer's can be like.

But her situation is horrifying. The video simply and elegantly shows viewers what it really means to have Alzheimer's. (You can see the video by searching the web for both "Volandes" and "dementia video.") When Volandes tested his video in a patient population, he found that it significantly reduced people's desires to receive aggressive care should they end up with end-stage dementia. A few minutes with his video and their minds were made up. If they ever suffered from end-stage dementia, they no longer wanted CPR or antibiotics or hospitalization. If they experienced a life-threatening illness, they now just wanted to be made comfortable so they could die in peace.

Volandes's video improves people's decision making by giving them a more accurate picture of life with Alzheimer's. But would Johnson's video do the same for colostomy? Alzheimer's is a terrible condition to imagine but an even worse condition to experience. People underestimate how bad life with Alzheimer's can be. The video shows the reality of Alzheimer's and therefore improves patients' decision making. By contrast, people typically overestimate how bad it would be to experience a colostomy. Johnson's video, like Volandes's, is very tastefully done. It shows that having a colostomy isn't necessarily a big deal, with Johnson's casual demeanor and healthy appearance potentially destigmatizing the condition. But all that tastefulness has to compete with a very powerful emotion. The people I have shown Johnson's video to almost always react with shock the first time they catch sight of his stoma. Many look away. Others look on in horror. Does Johnson's video elicit so much disgust that it unintentionally makes people think worse of life with a colostomy?

By now you know how I will answer this question. With the help of Andrea Angott, I conducted a simple experiment. We described what life with a colostomy was like to one group of people, including a detailed description of what colostomy patients must do to change their colostomy bags, and asked them what they thought their life would be like in similar circumstances. They weren't so keen on life with a colostomy. To another group of people we not only provided a description of life with a colostomy but also included Johnson's video. On average, this second group of people was more likely to believe that they could emotionally adapt to life with a colostomy. The video worked just as Johnson had intended. It minimized their fears about living with a colostomy.

The lesson of this research is not that videos necessarily improve people's ability to imagine unfamiliar health states. It is that the people designing decision aids can't figure out the best way to help patients make decisions unless they run experiments. They can't count on well-intentioned decision aids to lead patients to the right decision. Instead, they need to test the individual components of that decision aid to see how they influence patients' beliefs and judgments.

The lesson for patients is less straightforward. Those of you facing health-care decisions should not rush out to find explicit videos to inform your choice. I doubt, for instance, that a video of open-heart surgery is going to help you decide whether you need such an operation. Nevertheless, I'd guess that most patients would make better decisions if they had a concrete visualization of how their lives would be affected by their choice. Hearing from people who've "been there" is probably a good place to start. And you can expect an increasing number of decision aids to become available that provide such concrete images.

SHARED DECISION MAKING IS ABOUT BEHAVIOR CHANGE

In its infancy, the patient-empowerment revolution was correctly focused on power, on wresting decision-making authority from the exclusive grip of physicians. The power struggle was fought out in courts and debated in medical journals, with patients winning most of the major battles. But once the revolution left the domain of courts and journals and entered into medical clinics, the new power-sharing arrangement didn't work out as well as people had hoped. It didn't work because patients lacked knowledge; as long as doctors controlled the facts, patients could not be truly empowered.

Now, with the advent of decision aids, patients have access to the information they need in order to participate in their decisions, information increasingly provided to them in manners informed by the latest advances in behavioral science. With luck and hard work, we can hope such decision aids will soon become a standard part of clinical care. We are doing a disservice right now by letting so many patients struggle through hard choices without the help of a decision aid.

However, the goals of the revolution won't be reached simply by disseminating decision aids more widely. Informed patients are in a better position to partner with physicians than uninformed patients. But knowledge on its own won't inevitably lead to shared decision making. To fully equip patients for a partnership role we also need to prepare them for the often-challenging job of interacting successfully with their doctors.

ELEVEN

Coaching Patients to Be Partners

The year was 1992 and the Joint National Committee on Prevention, Detection, Evaluation, and Treatment of High Blood Pressure had just published its fifth report on the best way to—well, their name says it: prevent, detect, evaluate, and treat high blood pressure. The JNC5 report, as it was called, received a lot of attention in the medical community for the strong advice it gave doctors about how to treat patients with "uncomplicated hypertension"—patients who had moderately elevated blood pressure and no other major medical problems. I was a bioethics fellow at the University of Pittsburgh when the guidelines were published, and I remember being struck by how definitively the committee had promoted inexpensive generic blood pressure medicines over the newfangled alternatives, which had seduced most of us internists by then. At that time, many of us were scribbling names of calcium blockers like Cardizem and Procardia onto prescription pads faster than a new homeowner making her way through a stack of mortgage forms. The only thing slowing us down in prescribing calcium channel blockers was our temptation to prescribe another new class of drugs, ACE inhibitors like Prinivil and Vasotec, drugs whose names were scattered around our clinic work spaces on Post-it notes and pens given to us by attractive (always attractive!) sales representatives eager to convince us of the merits of

their products. Nowhere in our offices would you have found promotional materials espousing the benefits of generic blood pressure
medicines. No sales representatives dropped by our offices to tell us
about the wonders of hydrochlorothiazide, a water pill costing a few
cents per day, or to give us gifts adorned with the names of generic
beta blockers like atenolol. There wasn't enough money to be made
selling these drugs to justify expensive promotional campaigns.

No surprise then that in the years preceding JNC5, use of generic
water pills and beta blockers had declined significantly. The JNC
tried to combat this decline by shining a bright light on all of the
medical evidence supporting the superiority of generic medications.
Rigorous clinical trials had proven that drugs like hydrochlorothiazide and atenolol significantly reduced the risk of heart attacks and
strokes. The same couldn't then be said for calcium blockers and ACE
inhibitors. After summarizing the evidence, the JNC made a clear
recommendation: patients with uncomplicated hypertension should
be given water pills and beta blockers before being given these newer
drugs.

Yet data on prescribing patterns showed that doctors weren't
changing their behavior. Some were unaware of the JNC guidelines.
Others were so enthralled by the new drugs, and so used to dashing
their names off on their prescription pads, that they couldn't change
their ways, or didn't want to go through the hassle of switching patients from one drug to another, a switch that would not only take
time to explain but also might cause patients to experience uncontrolled blood pressure for a while. That didn't seem like a boat worth
rocking.

The result of this stubborn reluctance to change concerned me
greatly at the time. I was worried that patients were being exposed
to unnecessarily high risks of stroke and heart attack. And I was
bothered that they were also being subjected to an avoidable expense.
Generic medications were both effective and cheap, costing only pen-

nies a day. Calcium blockers and ACE inhibitors, on the other hand, cost several dollars a day, and a lot of that money came out of patients' pockets.

It was clear to me that patients faced a choice: cheap, safe, proven medications versus expensive but unproven ones. The choice seemed obvious. But of course a choice isn't a choice if you're not given a choice. Many patients taking these calcium blockers and ACE inhibitors were simply taking whatever drug their doctor had prescribed for them.

As a physician training in bioethics, I knew this was a choice patients ought to be involved in. Inspired by the decision-aid movement, I decided to develop an educational brochure that would convince patients to talk about the cost of their blood pressure medications with their doctors.

My plan was simple. I found an insurance company willing to let me introduce myself to patients who were receiving these expensive new drugs. I planned to ask for their permission to tape-record their next doctor visit. Then, when the patients arrived for their clinic appointments, I would provide half of them—selected at random—with my brochure.

While concocting my study, I met with my fellowship director, Dr. Wishwa Kapoor, a highly accomplished physician and brilliant researcher. Kapoor warned me that I was in over my head. "You haven't pilot-tested your intervention," he told me, "and you haven't conducted focus groups of patients or physicians to identify barriers to discussing the costs of blood pressure medication." He went on to correctly point out that I hadn't grounded my intervention in any theory of behavior change; nor had I decided how I would analyze what would inevitably be very complicated data—pharmacy records, patient questionnaires, and tape-recorded conversations. "This sounds like a five-year, two-million-dollar federal grant, Peter, and you haven't published a single paper in your career. You need to slow down."

I didn't. I plowed ahead and ran my study. I contacted the first half-dozen patients, all of whom were willing to take part in my study. I handed three of them the pamphlet in the clinic waiting room and turned on the tape recorder when they walked in to see their doctor. Then I went home to my apartment and listened to the first few audiotapes.

In none of them did any of the patients make a single mention of the high cost of their blood pressure drugs. I was shocked. My pamphlet had shown them how to save money—hundreds of dollars per year—by switching to generic medicines. It had explained in simple English that the drugs would probably improve their health. Yet patients weren't asking their doctors to consider switching them to such medicines? I had naïvely assumed that the only thing standing between these patients and affordable medicines was knowledge, that the truth would set them free. It hadn't occurred to me that these patients had longstanding, trusting relationships with their primary care physicians; that they might believe the newer, more expensive drugs were better than generic ones; or that some would feel embarrassed to bring up the topic with their doctors, as if questioning their doctors' judgment.

I still believe that patients need information about their health-care alternatives, including the financial cost, in order to receive the medical care they need and deserve. But I no longer believe that information is enough.

The idea of empowering patients through information is so appealing. We live in an age of information, after all. Having learned how to transform sights, sounds, and ideas into zeros and ones, we now stream that information across electrical outlets, radio waves, and cell towers to our laptops and hip pockets. Information is at our fingertips everywhere we wander. Whole economies thrive or struggle depending on whether they embrace this information age. Autocracies stand or topple depending on their ability to control information. In such an age, it hardly comes as a surprise that experts would believe that the key to patient empowerment is information. If the imbalance in power and pay between executives and laborers results at least in part from differences in their ability to process information, if the difference between first-world and third-world countries can be attributed to whether their economies are focused on information, then surely the huge chasm that separates doctors and patients, that causes patients to depend on their physicians for advice and guidance even when their own preferences ought to determine the best course of therapy—well, surely that chasm is best bridged with information. The informed patient will be an empowered decision maker. Or so the theory goes.

So much for theory.

I've already shown why decision aids, to reach their potential, need to incorporate insights from behavioral science in order to avoid unduly influencing patients' choices. My failed blood pressure experiment reveals another problem that information enthusiasts need to contend with if they hope to improve medical decision making: Preferences won't play their deserved role in patients' choices if these same patients remain hidden behind a wall of silence.

QUIET CONCERNS

By now, I have written enough about localized prostate cancer in this book that you probably know more about this disease than the typical man does when he arrives in his urologist's office and is told that "three out of twelve core biopsies" show cancer. You know that localized prostate cancer is not likely to be fatal. You have already learned that the patient will face a choice between watchful waiting, radiation, and surgery.

But those patients whose conversations I quoted in earlier chapters? All those men who sat silently through those incomprehensible urology soliloquies? You probably don't know as much about localized prostate cancer as they did at the time, because each of those men had been given a decision aid before meeting with their urologist. They knew the basics about their disease. They knew about their three treatment choices and the odds of experiencing side effects from each of those alternatives. They understood that localized prostate cancer is generally a slow-growing cancer. But they didn't know the specifics. They didn't know exactly which stage of localized cancer they had or whether their particular situation—their health history, for example—altered the risk–benefit ratio of any of their alternatives. The clinic visit was a chance for them to ask questions and an opportunity to talk with their doctor about their concerns. But most of them did very little talking, and few asked questions. Once again, I was listening to interactions in which informed patients sat passively while their doctors dominated the conversation.

Unlike my earlier study of blood pressure medicines, however, I wasn't caught off guard this time. My colleagues and I had pilot-tested our intervention. We had even acquired one of those hefty five-year grants I had earlier deemed unnecessary. One of the goals of our research was to document just how active or passive patients would be in this circumstance. In addition, we used this study to design an intervention that would help patients take a more active role in their decision.

I will tell you more about that intervention later but, for now, imagine yourself as one of those patients. You have learned about prostate cancer, but until you walked into that office, you hadn't learned that you had been diagnosed with this illness. Prior to the visit, you knew that localized prostate cancer was not a death sentence, but you didn't know that, after the doctor delivered the bad news, your heart rate would double and your mind would race while your urologist spouted off a detailed breakdown of your Gleason score in language very different from the plain-language decision aid you had read before the appointment. You didn't realize that you would want to ask questions but, before you could get a word in edgewise, your urologist would be two paragraphs further into his elaborate presentation, the questions now forgotten. You had no idea that you would feel guilty even contemplating interrupting him to request clarification.

Decision aids do a great job of informing patients about their illnesses. But they often do very little to prepare patients for how to take an active role in conversations with their doctors. Would patients benefit from being more active? Or would the responsibility only burden them? To begin getting answers to these questions, we need to make a quick visit to a nursing home.

AN IDEA BLOOMS

In the early 1970s, St. Bonaventure's (a pseudonym) was one of the finest nursing homes in Connecticut, with excellent nurse-to-patient ratios and state-of-the-art facilities. Yet its residents were not exactly thriving. Old and frail, most of them were steadily declining toward their inevitable ends. As their muscles weakened, residents would retreat to their rooms over the months and years of their stay, no longer strong enough to attend movies or bingo contests. Eventually they would become bedridden, the end now almost something to look forward to.

Judith Rodin and Ellen Langer didn't think these nursing home residents should have to decline so quickly. A resident's withdrawal from nursing home life didn't need to be so inevitable. Rodin and Langer's training in social psychology convinced them that if these residents had more control over their own lives, their decline might be slowed. So they convinced St. Bonaventure's to let them conduct a randomized trial of a simple intervention, one that would reframe the residents' nursing home experiences so they would take active control of their own lives.

They ran a simple experiment. The nursing home staff spoke with half the residents about what they could expect from living in the nursing home, emphasizing what nursing home employees would do to care for their needs. Want the furniture rearranged in your room? The nursing home staff would do that for them, if asked. ("We want your rooms to be as nice as they can be, and we've tried to make them that way for you.") Want to go to a movie? No problem. In fact, half of the residents would be assigned to Friday night movie viewing and the remainder to Thursday. ("We'll let you know later which day you're scheduled to see it.") The staff then concluded by giving each resident a plant and informing them that nursing home employees would make sure to water and care for the plant every day.

The remaining residents, the intervention group, were also told that they could have their furniture rearranged, but this time the staff emphasized that this would only happen if the residents took the initiative to call the staff for help. ("You should be deciding how you want your rooms to be arranged—whether you want it to be as it is or whether you want the staff to help you rearrange the furniture.") These residents were also informed that the nursing home screened movies on Thursday and Friday nights, but they were told it was up to *them* to decide which night they wanted to attend. ("You should decide which night you'd like to go, if you choose to see it at all.") And like the others, they were given plants to put into their rooms, but with a reminder that it was *their* responsibility to water and care for their plants each day if they wanted the plants to survive.

What happened to these two groups of nursing home residents stands as one of the most amazing experimental results in the history of social psychology. The intervention group blossomed in the presence of their newfound responsibilities. When the nursing home scheduled group activities, they were five to ten times more likely to attend than other residents. Movie night became a regular part of their lives, while the other group, no longer responsible for choosing which night to go, were more likely to stay in their rooms. Plus, those in the intervention group were significantly happier than other residents. Their sense of responsibility for their lives caused them to emotionally thrive. Even more amazingly, when Rodin and Langer checked on the nursing home residents eighteen months later—a year and a half after their simple, hour-long intervention—they discovered that the intervention group had experienced a 50 percent reduction in mortality. That's right, in mortality! Empowered to take control over tiny parts of their lives, they had thrived beyond anyone's expectations.

When Jack Wennberg discovered variations in hysterectomy rates, he thought it was time to empower patients. When Rodin and Langer discovered rapid declines in the health and well-being of nursing home residents, they decided to test whether empowering these residents would improve their lives. It seems that empowerment was the theme of the day. The late '60s and early '70s were a time, as we have seen, when people across the United States and Europe were fighting to have more power, more control over their lives. It was not shocking, then, that Wennberg and Rodin and Langer would independently arrive at the idea that laypeople needed to be empowered to thrive.

But what would it take to empower patients in medical clinics? The answer to that question was discovered by a pair of researchers from RAND who had set out to measure the quality of medical care.

YOUR SUGAR OR YOUR LIFE

Sheldon Greenfield was a physician who worked at both RAND and UCLA. Sherrie Kaplan was a graduate student at the UCLA School of Public Health. They met at RAND in 1973 when the two were pulled into a research project RAND leaders believed would inform the federal government's efforts to reform the U.S. health-care system.

At the time, it looked like President Nixon was ready to provide health insurance to the U.S. population. "Early last year," he communicated in a special message to Congress, "I directed the Secretary of

Health, Education, and Welfare to prepare a new and improved plan for comprehensive health insurance." (To his other sins, I guess, we have to now acknowledge that Richard Nixon was a socialist!) Researchers at RAND were frantically scrambling to complete projects that would help the government craft successful legislation. Greenfield and Kaplan were part of a team tasked with figuring out ways a government-run health-care system could determine whether it was providing high-quality care to its patients.

As Kaplan tells the story, the research team developed a series of algorithms that clinical coders could use to evaluate quality of care. For example, an algorithm might indicate that if a patient presents with X, then the doctor should do either Y or Z. Using the algorithm, coders could flag instances when doctors failed to do either Y or Z as possible examples of inappropriate care. Greenfield and Kaplan worked diligently to make it easy for the coders, none of whom were physicians, to nevertheless make relatively accurate judgments about the quality of care physicians were providing.

Whether or not the algorithms truly captured the complexities of medical care is a debatable topic, but the ease of using the algorithms was unquestionable. The algorithms were so simple to use, so intuitive that the nurse-practitioners using the algorithms would find themselves describing the clinical rules to friends at cocktail parties. And the laypeople conversing with the nurse-practitioners would get excited about the topic. "Oh, that's what the doctors are supposed to do. Fascinating. But what would they need to do if . . . ?"

Kaplan learned about all these cocktail conversations and it gave her an idea: "If the algorithms are this easy to understand and use, why don't we give them to patients?"

Greenfield and Kaplan, in one of their early studies, decided to get diabetes patients more involved in their medical care by teaching them some of the algorithms. Chronic diseases like diabetes require patients to make repeated choices, allowing them to try out different alternatives over time to see what works best. People with diabetes face many choices about how best to treat their disease, but few of the choices are irreversible. If they aren't sure whether they'll be able to tolerate insulin injections, for example, they can try injections for a couple of weeks to see how they feel. If they aren't sure that life on a strict diet will be worth living, they can try out the diet for a while and see whether the drop in their blood sugar is gratifying enough to make up for having to live with hunger pangs.

This ability to try out choices ought to be empowering for patients, as they are no longer dependent on physicians to describe their alternatives. Even more empowering should be the control patients have over many aspects of their treatment. If a doctor prescribes a diabetes pill that makes a patient feel bad, that patient can decide not to take the pill. If a doctor "orders" a patient to check her blood sugars three times a day, to avoid all desserts, and to exercise five times a week— well, that patient has the final say in all these matters. If she wants to skip the gym to make a trip to Dunkin' Donuts, the physician is powerless to intervene. Because people typically live with diabetes for so many years, most diabetic patients become experts in their disease: virtuosos at pricking their fingers to assess their blood sugar, painfully familiar with what it feels like to watch calories, masters of knowing what happens to their sugar readings when they don't watch their calories. More than anything, they come to learn that it is *they* who are in charge of their illness.

Yet many people with diabetes don't feel empowered by their illness. Many don't even take the time to fully grasp the pros and cons of bringing their blood sugar under control. So they hover between paradigms. Despite being the ones who decide each morning whether to take their pills, they too often become passive in the presence of their doctors.

Greenfield and Kaplan knew it didn't have to be this way. They knew that with the right information and, more importantly, with some coaching as to how to be more active in their care, these patients could get a better handle on their diabetes. Greenfield and Kaplan arranged for each patient to meet with a research assistant before their appointment. The research assistant helped each patient identify the kinds of health decisions he or she would have to make during the appointment, such as which diabetes medications to take and whether to try a new diet. The research assistant also gave each patient a brief tutorial on how to negotiate with their doctor, a ten-minute primer on how to discuss treatment preferences. Finally, the research assistant coached each patient about what to do if they encountered obstacles.

The whole session took twenty minutes, a blink of an eye compared to the hours these patients had spent in medical clinics over the course of their lives. Nevertheless, the brief intervention had a huge effect on patients. When the doctors arrived in the office, the patients began asking more questions, no longer letting doctors dominate the conversation. The effect of the intervention wasn't limited to the clinical appointment; when the patients returned to the clinic several months later, they had substantially lower blood sugars, with reductions in glucose that rivaled those brought about by the strongest available pills.

Greenfield and Kaplan's intervention didn't work simply by increasing patients' knowledge of their diabetes. It didn't work by increasing how long patients spent talking with their physicians. It worked the same way those nursing home plants worked—by empowering patients to take charge of their lives. Before the intervention, most patients felt that they couldn't do much about their diabetes, other than take whatever medicines their doctors prescribed. Their disease was like a nursing home plant under the care of someone else. But after Greenfield and Kaplan's intervention, they felt activated. They no longer felt overwhelmed by either their doctors or their blood sugar readings—that damn diabetes was now their responsibility!

In the past few decades, behavioral scientists have developed several effective ways in which to engage patients more actively in their medical care. The research shows that patients are better at engaging in their medical care when they receive concrete, vivid examples of how to interact with their doctors. Telling a patient that "it's your decision to make" doesn't give patients a concrete image of what they can do to get more involved in their decisions. Anyone even a bit shy about speaking up in front of their doctor won't overcome their fear with a simple exhortation to "ask lots of questions." And keep in mind, as Kaplan colorfully pointed out to me, "It's hard to be assertive when you're naked." The best interventions give patients examples of how to talk to doctors and even provide them with a chance to practice such behaviors.

That's why, when Angie Fagerlin and I listened to our prostate cancer recordings, we knew we needed to supplement our decision aid with a coaching tool. We created a DVD designed to help men visualize their upcoming urology appointment. We give men the DVD before their urology appointment, so they will be prepared to discuss treatment alternatives should their biopsy reveal cancer. The DVD begins with a video clip of a urologist telling a man that he has prostate cancer. A narrator then explains that the doctor and patient are actors reenacting encounters between urologists and prostate cancer patients. The DVD cuts back and forth between urology clinic reenactments and the narrator. One scene shows a urologist providing a long and confusing description of a patient's Gleason score while the patient sits silently. The narrator then explains what is happening in the encounter and gives suggestions about how patients can take action to improve the encounter, followed by scenes showing the patient using each of these techniques. The DVD coaches patients on how to politely assert themselves, within the context of a realistic encounter. It helps patients concretely visualize their upcoming visit. It even helps patients understand what's going on in their doctors' minds. After showing a clip of the urologist telling his patient he has

cancer, for instance, the DVD cuts to an interview with the actor playing the role of the patient. "After the doctor told me I had cancer," the
patient says, "the next few minutes felt like a blur." The DVD helps
patients anticipate how they will feel and prepares them for how this
will influence the encounter. The narrator explains that "all the numbers can be confusing and overwhelming" and then gives the patient
examples of how they can slow down the conversation. Reenactments
of the scene follow, with the patient trying different strategies to
help the doctor communicate more effectively. A scene in which the
patient nods along, pretending to understand, is followed by one in
which the patient doesn't hesitate to furrow his brow. A scene where
the patient passively attempts to absorb the onslaught of information
is followed by several in which the patient either gently interrupts the
doctor or his spouse asks the doctor to slow down so that she can take
notes.

The DVD even helps patients understand their doctors better. At
one point the narrator asks the viewer to "imagine how the doctor
probably feels at this time. It's not easy to give patients bad news. We
think that may explain why some doctors move very quickly from
breaking the bad news right into the long and technical discussions of
a patient's diagnosis." By revealing the humanity of the physician—
the weakness, the emotional fragility—we hope to bring doctors and
patients closer together, so they can communicate better.

Our DVD uses insights from behavioral science research to help
prepare patients for their upcoming visits. We address people's
thoughts and emotions while helping them visualize what to expect
in their visit. We even give patients suggestions about how to influence the course of the encounter. In effect, our DVD acts like a communication coach.

But there is a problem. Not all decisions are common enough and
predictable enough in their clinical content to warrant the filming of
a disease-specific DVD. Fortunately, there's a way to overcome this

problem. Decision-making experts at some of the world's best medical centers are starting to team patients with decision coaches!

THERE'S NO "I" IN COACH

Renee Beaumont was proof that fifty-two is the new thirty-two. The year was 2007 and Beaumont laughed at the thought the she was middle-aged, finding the energy after teaching high school science during the day to dance at her local studio for three or four hours each night. Not casual dancing either, but en pointe ballet. Strangers would not have guessed she was in her early fifties. Even her body seemed to have been duped, since she hadn't even experienced the first signs of menopause.

Things changed rapidly, however, when the follow-up mammogram she'd been putting off for six years abruptly brought her back to reality. She had a 5 cm mass in her right breast, a growth the size of a ripe plum. Her primary care physician sent her to meet with a breast surgeon. "She walked into the room," Beaumont told me, "reviewed the mammogram and said, almost robotically, 'Okay, it's a cancer.' I was completely shocked. I thought it would be a cyst, because I'd had those before. But then she kept right on talking, and next thing I know she was telling me I needed a biopsy right away."

Beaumont's biopsy confirmed the surgeon's suspicions, so Beaumont was soon back in the doctor's office, this time receiving instructions for an urgent procedure. "You need a mastectomy," the surgeon told her. "I can schedule you for next week, which means we can get you treated before I head out on vacation. Otherwise we'll have to wait two more weeks, and I don't want to delay that long."

Beaumont was overwhelmed with fear and shock—fear that she'd not live to see her fifty-third birthday; shock that her dancer's body, so much a part of her self-identity, had now betrayed her. She was terrified that her disease was progressing at such a rapid pace that she couldn't even wait a couple of weeks for surgery. Yet despite her emotional state, Beaumont rejected her doctor's recommendation. She didn't schedule a surgery date right away. She told the surgeon she needed "more time to think."

True to her word, Beaumont did a lot of thinking over the next few days. And crying. She huddled together with friends and family to commiserate over her situation. She also began educating herself about her treatment options. The biopsy had shown that her tumor was an example of what doctors call DCIS—ductal carcinoma in situ. Reading up on this condition, Beaumont discovered that DCIS typically behaves more like a pre-cancer than a full-blown cancer. Although sometimes DCIS progresses to invasive cancer, other times it is more indolent, neither expanding locally nor spreading to distant organs. Some experts even question whether DCIS tumors require any kind of active therapy. The urgent mastectomy recommendation she had received, in other words, was not supported by rigorous medical evidence.

Yet, of the more than 5,000 women diagnosed with DCIS in the United States every year, the vast majority of them end up getting surgery. They go under the knife even though no study has shown that such aggressiveness prolongs their lives. Beaumont hated the thought of surgery, and her reading proved to her satisfaction that, at a minimum, she had time to get a second opinion.

After a bit of haggling, Beaumont received permission from her insurance company to see a surgeon at the University of California, San Francisco, an institution not on the insurance company's list of providers. She was told she could get an opinion at UCSF but no operation. That meant, if she decided to undergo the procedure, she'd need to return to her first surgeon.

The UCSF surgeon was very pleasant if a bit "aristocratic," as Beaumont described her to me. The surgeon answered Beaumont's questions with methodical thoroughness. And Beaumont had plenty of questions: "At one point in the visit I said, 'I have just one more question,' to which the surgeon replied, 'You've been saying that for twenty minutes!'"

Throughout the conversation, the UCSF surgeon was adamant that Beaumont's tumor required treatment. "You need a mastectomy," she said. "Would lumpectomy be an option?" Beaumont asked. "No, it wouldn't. If I try a wide-angle incision [to preserve the rest of the right breast] it would be horribly misshapen." Beaumont was too disgusted by the thought of maiming her body to accept this recommendation. In frustration, she blurted out a defiant question: "Well, what if I just don't do anything?" The surgeon's face suddenly broke out into a grin. "Well, . . . you *could* do that. Yes. That's an option."

Then the surgeon described a clinical trial Beaumont could enter if she was willing to forgo surgery for the time being. If she chose to enroll in the trial, Beaumont would start by taking tamoxifen for a few months. Beaumont leapt at the opportunity. After all, anything was better than surgery.

By now it should be obvious that Renee Beaumont did not need a decision aid or an accompanying DVD to be an active participant in her health-care decisions. Her natural tenacity and her science background combined to give her the confidence to challenge both of her surgeons. It didn't hurt that she also possessed a strong and consistent desire to avoid mastectomy. But the next chapter of Beaumont's story left her very much in need of decision-making assistance.

Beaumont dutifully took her tamoxifen tablets for three months and received promising results—follow-up tests showed that her tumor hadn't grown any larger. She was ecstatic to learn the news. But the UCSF surgeon was less impressed, pointing out that the tumor hadn't shrunk on the medication, which meant she still had a ping-pong-ball-size mass in her breast: "We need to get this cancer out of you." Once again Beaumont found herself in conflict with a surgeon who was eager for her to undergo a mastectomy. Almost at the point of despair now, Beaumont didn't know what to do. That's when she got a call from a decision coach.

Beaumont's coach was a premedical student from UCSF. The student was volunteering in UCSF's Decision Services program, a decision coaching resource established by Jeff Belkora in 2003. Belkora is a systems engineer at UCSF who created an innovative approach to coaching that paired patients with students—people studying medicine, nursing, social work, or other health-related professions. Belkora's team trained these students to help patients communicate with their physicians and sort through their medical options.

Beaumont's first interaction with her decision coach was on the telephone. The coach listened while Beaumont told her story and then asked Beaumont what questions she still felt her surgeon hadn't answered. Beaumont brought up a few points of concern. But the coach wasn't satisfied. The questions were confusing. So Beaumont rephrased the questions. Eventually the coach understood what she wanted. "You want to know about active surveillance," she said. It suddenly dawned on Beaumont that part of her difficulty communicating with her doctors was that she did not know how to convey her concerns to them in a language they would understand. Thanks to the help of the coach, Beaumont now had a way to translate her questions and concerns into medical language.

There is plenty of irony in Beaumont's situation. So often, as we have seen, physicians forget how to communicate to patients in a language that patients understand. Beaumont's experience proves that this problem runs in both directions. The UCSF Decision Services program teaches patients enough medical language to better communicate with their physicians. Often this means helping patients rehearse and revise their questions until they are concrete instead of amorphous. "A patient might start with a vague concern, such as a fear of side effects," Belkora told me. "The coaches are trained to help them clarify this concern. 'What are you afraid of? What have you read?' a coach might say and then the patient might say they are afraid the treatment will cause another cancer. At that point, the coach will usually work with the patent to write down their concern in the form of a question they can ask their doctor."

When the coach accompanied Beaumont to her next appointment, another benefit of the decision service became immediately apparent. "I didn't have to take notes," Beaumont told me excitedly. "I could finally concentrate on what the doctor was saying." The coach took notes at each of Beaumont's appointments. The notes were a great help to Beaumont because they tersely summarized the major topics her doctor discussed. Beaumont also discovered that the coach helped her understand the clinical situation better. And most importantly, thanks to the presence of the coach, Beaumont felt even more confident about expressing her opinions to her doctor. The surgeon had already acknowledged in previous visits that the best way to treat DCIS was controversial. But the surgeon had always returned to the need for surgery, arguing that it was "better to be safe than sorry." Beaumont hadn't found the right way to tell the surgeon that it wasn't lack of safety that would make her sorry. She was mainly worried about living with the idea that she had had her breast removed unnecessarily. Now that the coach had helped her understand the medical evidence better and had given her the opportunity to practice expressing her concerns, she was more confident in communicating her unique preferences to the surgeon.

Thanks to the decision-coaching program, Beaumont was able to convince her surgeon to monitor her tumor without having to spend the majority of each appointment arguing about the need for a mastectomy. In 2009, Beaumont was even able to avoid this operation despite the fact that her surveillance testing revealed an area within her tumor that had acquired a few new flecks of calcium, a signal (later confirmed by biopsy) that the tumor had become more aggressive. With this turn for the worse, the surgeon pushed once again for a mastectomy but, thanks to the help of the coach, Beaumont was prepared to push back. "Why not just remove the part within the tumor that looks more aggressive?" she asked. The surgeon hadn't heard of anyone taking out an invasive cancer while leaving the surrounding DCIS tumor alone. But she couldn't entirely dismiss the idea. "We don't know it won't help you," she told Beaumont. Translated into clearer English, that meant it might just work!

Two and a half years later, Beaumont's DCIS tumor remains quiescent in her right breast. She continues to pursue a program of active surveillance. And she still dances.

THE KEY TO PATIENT EMPOWERMENT

I have now described a range of interventions that attempt to empower patients with knowledge about their health-care alternatives and provide them with the tools to better assert themselves when interacting with their doctors. I've described decision aids—web-based or video programs designed to help patients understand their health-care alternatives for a wide range of medical situations. You can find up-to-date lists of decision aids at the University of Ottawa's website (decisionaid.ohri.ca/), thanks to the pioneering efforts of a nurse researcher named Annette O'Connor. You should also check out the website of the Informed Medical Decisions Foundation (IMDF), the organization started by Jack Wennberg's team (www.informedmedical decisions.org).

I've described efforts by behavioral scientists like me to help decision-aid developers design decision aids in ways that won't accidentally bias patients' choices. Teams of experts from around the world are working together to incorporate these behavioral insights into decision aids. The University of Ottawa and IMDF websites list the best available decision aids. If you have an important decision to make, make an effort to get ahold of a decision aid.

And I've described Jeff Belkora's decision-coaching service at UCSF. I wish I could say such services were sprouting up all over the place. But at the time I was finishing this book, there weren't more than a few such services I'd become aware of. Nevertheless, you can begin to approximate Belkora's approach. If you are being cared for in an academic medical center, grab as much of the medical or nursing students' time as you can. If you're going to a doctor's appointment, bring along someone to take notes or bring along a tape recorder.

The existence of these interventions is good news for all of us, because medical decisions are an inevitable part of each of our lives. Whether you someday have to decide about antibiotics for a sore throat or open-heart surgery for a failing aortic valve, your chance of being powerless to partner in the decision, of being too uninformed to weigh the pros and cons of your alternatives, is smaller now than it has ever been, because the shared decision-making interventions I have talked about are on the rise.

For all the promise of these new interventions, however, patients still face a major challenge. The modern health-care system and the physicians who practice within it are not necessarily prepared to work with prepared patients. To understand the magnitude of this challenge, we need to see what can happen when a knowledgeable and assertive patient confronts a series of doctors who aren't ready to share the decision-making burden.

PART IV

Learning to Share

TWELVE

The Limits of Patient Empowerment

In the spring of 2011 Paula Greeno lay anesthetized on an operating room table, her left breast splayed open where the surgeon had removed a small cancer. They were at the point in the operation when the surgeon would busy himself either closing the wound, sewing the cleaved tissues back together and finishing the procedure, or expanding the operation by opening the wound up a bit more so he could remove lymph nodes from her armpit. But the surgeon was neither closing nor opening. In fact, he wasn't anywhere to be seen. He had left the operating room to speak with Greeno's husband about an important decision.

"I'm sorry to say that one of the two lymph nodes we removed from Paula's axilla [her armpit] was positive for metastatic cancer, a one-centimeter mass visible on the frozen section."

"Oh," the husband replied, the news hitting him like a helmet-to-helmet tackle.

"That means we have to decide whether to remove more lymph nodes," the surgeon continued. "We could do that right now, but if that's not necessarily what she would want, we can finish up the operation and talk to her when she wakes up, then decide whether to go back for those lymph nodes next week."

"In another operation?"

"Yes."

"But . . ."

"What do you think Paula would want?"

Her husband sat silently befuddled. Why, he wondered, hadn't they discussed this important decision before the operation began, while Paula was awake and could express her opinion? Why had they not taken time to consider the pros and cons of lymph node dissection before beginning the surgery? Flooded with anger, confusion, and panic (his wife was still in the operating room and he needed to make up his mind!), and overwhelmed by a tremendous sense of responsibility, he considered the options. Nothing leading up to that moment had hinted at the possibility that he could be playing the role of Gerald Ford, deciding what to do about his wife's breast cancer while she lay sleeping on an operating room table. The year was 2011, after all, not 1975. He and his wife had worked hard to educate themselves about her treatment decisions, had even reviewed a breast cancer decision aid before the operation. What's more, the husband thought of himself as a bit of a medical decision-making expert. He had been confident that he and his wife had done everything humanly possible to make decisions together—together as a couple and together with their surgeon. Yet somehow he was being forced to make a decision no husband should have to make.

Can you imagine what it felt like to be put into this position? I can, because that husband was me.

It is not possible for a patient and spouse to have been more empowered than Paula and I were in the days leading up to her surgery. From the time of Paula's diagnosis, we had both played an incredibly active role in her treatment decisions. We'd educated ourselves about the latest medical research, even spoke with colleagues across the country who were experts in breast cancer diagnosis and treatment. We believed we had asserted ourselves well enough during Paula's medical appointments to have sorted out all the details of her medical care.

Clearly we were wrong. We weren't as empowered as we'd thought. And now I sat there talking to Paula's surgeon, empowered to make a decision that Paula couldn't participate in. Despite my best efforts to partner with Paula in battling her illness, I'd found myself face-to-face with the limits of patient empowerment.

How could someone with my knowledge, confidence, and general decision-making expertise (and humility too!) end up in this situation? It all began with what I mistakenly believed to be a routine and unnecessary mammogram.

DEATH PANEL DEBATES AND SCREENING SQUABBLES

Legislators and White House staff were working around the clock, drafting what they hoped would be Barack Obama's signature piece of domestic legislation when the news hit—the United States Preventive Services Task Force (USPSTF) had published recommendations calling for women to delay their first mammogram until age fifty. It was the fall of 2009, and Democrats had already spent the summer fending off the notion that their health-reform legislation called for the creation of what Sarah Palin so colorfully characterized as "death panels" on her Facebook page that summer: "The America I know and love is not one in which my parents or my baby with Down Syndrome will have to stand in front of Obama's 'death panel' so his bureaucrats can decide, based on a subjective judgment of their 'level of productivity in society,' whether they are worthy of health care."

I followed the death panel and mammography controversies fairly closely when they happened. But almost a year and a half later, in the winter of 2010, I read even more widely about both controversies in preparation for an undergraduate course I was teaching on health-care policy, a class in which I spiced up otherwise dry topics like insurance reform by engaging students in ethical and political debates, complete with video clips from the town hall confrontations during which angry constituents had confronted Democratic legislators, complaining about their dangerous, death-promoting health-care bill. I reminded myself that my youngest students had been juniors in high school when the town hall meetings had occurred and probably had not been glued to *All Things Considered* podcasts. So I crafted a lecture on the politics of mammography. I put together some slides exploring the pros and cons of mammograms in forty-year-old women, so the students would have a feel for the science underlying the task force's recommendation. I laid out the benefits of mammograms for such women—these tests do save lives, after all, by identifying early cancers that can be slowed with treatment. And I laid out the risks: mammograms expose women to radiation, and they often identify suspicious shadows that lead to painful and potentially risky follow-up tests, like biopsies, tests that are usually benign—false positives, as we medical experts title them—false positives that create unnecessary fear and anxiety.

Later that winter, Paula told me she was scheduling a mammogram. With the USPSTF report still bouncing around in my head, I felt compelled to dissuade her. "You are only forty-four years old, and you had a normal mammogram just a year ago," I reminded her (as if a woman needs to be reminded about either her age or the last time her breasts were squeezed in a vise grip). "Your primary care physician is going overboard. Save yourself the trouble." I did not know then that Paula's primary care doctor had felt a lump in Paula's left breast. Paula was convinced it was a cyst, since her previous mammogram had revealed a cyst in the same general location. But she wanted to make sure and she didn't want me to feel undue alarm. So she told me she understood my concerns and then decided to go ahead with the mammogram.

A few days later I was at my office when Paula forwarded me an e-mail with her mammography report attached. I didn't look at it right away because I had to run to a meeting. That evening she asked me if I'd read it yet, in a manner that suggested that I'd better turn the answer into a yes right away, so I flipped open my iPad and opened the e-mail attachment while Paula waited expectantly for my reaction. After some introductory generalities, the report cut to the chase: "There is a 1.7 cm irregular mass with a spiculated margin in the left breast at six o'clock."

A jolt of fear shot through my body. I knew that most breast masses aren't cancer, but I also knew most masses aren't "spiculated," a word we doctors use when a mass contains long, jagged limbs, as if stretching beyond its normal boundaries. Spiculated masses look energetic and angry, not rounded and content like benign cysts. Reading frantically through the rest of the report, my eyes landed on the radiologist's terse summary of the situation: "The palpable mass is likely to be a cancer."

Shit.

Paula watched as I read the report and saw the upset look on my face. We exchanged a this-totally-sucks look, careful about what we vocalized, because our boys were reading quietly (for a change) on a nearby couch. We spoke sotto voce about the situation. I reminded her that most breast biopsies turn out to be negative, and that even if her biopsy showed cancer, it was going to be an *early,* very treatable cancer. Maybe (I told myself but not Paula) it would be a pseudo-cancer like DCIS, a cancer in name only but nothing, surely nothing that would threaten her health or, God forbid, shorten her lifespan. In effect, without any good evidence about what was happening to my wife's body and with a strong suspicion that her mass was a cancer, I started administering large doses of hope and optimism, as much to calm my own nerves as to calm Paula's.

THE FIRST BIG DECISION

The next few days were quite stressful, stuck as we were in the diagnostic limbo between the radiologist's suspicion of cancer and the pathologist's confirmation. The stress was always hardest on Paula at the end of the day. She'd lie in bed telling me she didn't want our children going to high school without a mom while I went into hope overdrive to counter her very real and understandable fears.

The biopsy did little to reduce our stress. Paula's mass was an invasive cancer, nothing as mild as the DCIS I had hoped for—crappy news, by any account. But there was also a bit of good news in the biopsy report: 100 percent of the cells had estrogen and progestin receptors on their surfaces. This meant that the growth of Paula's tumor depended heavily on being bathed in her hormones. Deprive the tumor of such hormones and it wouldn't grow as fast. That was a great prognostic sign. It was partly this combination of good and bad news that reinforced our stress levels, contributing to the feeling that we were still in limbo. But even more stressful was our realization that this new diagnosis meant we had an important decision to make.

We had to decide between mastectomy and lumpectomy. We had not yet met with a surgeon, but we knew enough about breast cancer to prepare ourselves for the appointment. Even though we were early in the decision process, Paula already had a strong preference for breast-conserving treatment, if that would be an option. She expressed that preference to her surgical oncologist when he called her to set up an appointment.

I know that sounds backward. Surgeons don't usually call up patients to set up appointments. But one of our friends, a famous breast cancer researcher, unbeknownst to us, had contacted the surgeon and asked him to take good care of her. The surgeon then very kindly and generously found time to fit Paula into his busy schedule.

Clearly our experience dealing with Paula's cancer is not typical. Most breast cancer patients and their partners aren't friends with breast cancer researchers. Most aren't as savvy about medical care as we were either. You know my background already. Paula's background complemented mine quite well in preparing us for her medical journey. I had met Paula in 1991, when she was an M.B.A. student at the University of Chicago. She'd entered business school with a goal of pursuing a finance degree but decided partway through her studies to switch to health-care management, feeling as if she could do more good for the world in health care than in finance. We met when she started attending ethics committee meetings at the University of Chicago hospital.

After graduating from business school, Paula worked her way up the health-care management ladder, not only learning the ins and outs of how medical centers function but also getting to know medical muckety-mucks from around the country. She had met and even battled with enough medical school department chairs and deans that she was no longer intimidated by physicians in white coats. During one stretch of time she helped a breast cancer clinic reorganize its outpatient facilities; in the process she even sat in on doctor–patient encounters to learn how the clinic worked.

Together, then, we possessed a combination of knowledge and confidence that few patients bring to their clinical encounters. And while our unusual backgrounds make our story atypical, they also make the details of our story that much more alarming. Paula's story is important because it demonstrates that even when empowered and activated patients confront important medical decisions, things don't always work out the way they should.

DR. FEELGOOD

I am an optimist by nature, so when Paula's biopsy revealed cancer, I kept telling myself it was a really early cancer, practically a non-cancer. Remove it and the threat would be gone. Indeed, when I began brushing up on breast cancer staging, my optimistic view seemed to be confirmed. According to the National Cancer Institute, the first factor that determines breast cancer stage is the size of the tumor, with tumors less than 2 cm being stage 1 (the best stage) and those larger being stage 2 (or staged higher, if there is evidence of spread). Paula's tumor was only 1.7 cm, according to the mammography report. Solidly within stage 1—phew!

We came into the surgeon's office already leaning toward lumpectomy but eager to hear what he had to say about the two alternatives. An impressive man, with more letters after his last name than I have in mine, he had already gone out of his way to accommodate Paula's busy schedule but nevertheless acted as if he had all day to talk with us about her diagnosis. Before going into any details of her treatment options, however, he needed to examine her.

Paula's tumor was on the underside of her left breast. He palpated the mass and remarked, offhandedly, that it felt a little bigger than 2 cm. He continued his exam while I began obsessing on his offhanded remark. Rationally speaking, I knew that the biological difference between a 1.7 cm mass and a 2.1 cm mass is insubstantial. I knew that blunt categories like staging systems draw sharp lines where none exist; these categories are primarily of use in research, so doctors can standardize the patients they recruit into clinical trials. If a new drug offers potential benefits to women with early breast cancer, doctors testing the drug need to decide what they mean by "early." They make arbitrary cutoffs and these cutoffs become stages.

Rationally speaking, I knew it didn't matter much whether Paula's tumor was slightly under or slightly over 2 cm, but I wasn't in a rational mood. The surgeon's offhanded remark struck me like a lightning bolt. I found myself wondering how he could have been so cavalier and insensitive to remark on the size of her tumor. He had the temerity to overrule Paula's radiology report and to declare that my wife's tumor was greater than 2 cm? That her cancer was stage 2? But he wasn't so irrational as to be hung up on tumor staging. If he had made any mistake in stating his belief about the size of Paula's tumor, it was in not realizing that I was irrationally obsessed with tumor staging.

I might have been far more educated about breast cancer than the typical person, but my education was quite uneven, giving me just enough knowledge to make wrong conclusions. One of the challenges of the new paradigm is that when patients inform themselves about their diagnoses before talking with their doctors—with decision aids or, more often, with visits to Internet sites—their education is incomplete. It comes with partial information and with a good deal of misinformation. These empowered patients then march into their doctors' offices thinking they know more than they know, while their doctors plow ahead unaware of what any given patient knows or believes.

Paula's surgeon wasn't worried about what I knew or didn't know. He was concerned about the location of Paula's tumor. He didn't think he'd be able to remove it and also achieve a good cosmetic outcome. Cosmetic appearance is often a significant problem for women with lumpectomies. In fact, a couple of years before Paula's diagnosis I had collaborated on a survey of breast cancer patients which revealed that many of these women are unhappy about the appearance of their lumpectomies. Many complain that their affected breasts are misshapen, with big indentations in the location where their cancers used to be. Others protest that their two breasts no longer match in size. Many are so bothered by breast asymmetry that they opt for plastic surgery to reshape their breasts.

Paula wondered whether there was a way to improve the cosmetic outcome of a lumpectomy. "If they need to remove a lot of breast tissue to get the cancer out, can they do a partial reconstruction to fill in the area? Perhaps a partial implant?" she asked. "No," the surgeon responded. "That's not an option."

We discussed the pros and cons of mastectomy and lumpectomy for a while longer, but soon the surgeon explained that we wouldn't be making a decision that day. "I'm concerned about some calcifications on your mammogram," he told Paula, "which might be trails of tumor. I want those biopsied. If there is cancer in any other part of your breast, you'll need a mastectomy."

Paula then asked the surgeon for his opinion on another aspect of her treatment: "Am I going to need chemo?"

"I'm not an oncologist," he replied, "so I prefer sticking to my specialty and letting the oncologists stick to theirs. But I'd have to say that, given your age and the size of the tumor, you have chemotherapy in your future."

We had come to Paula's first post-diagnosis appointment expecting to make a surgical decision, but the decision was put off for another day. We returned to the unsettling life of pre-decisional limbo and, for Paula, to the additional fear of chemotherapy.

BACK TO THE DECISION TREE

Women with early-stage breast cancer face a daunting number of treatment choices. The first choice, as we have seen, is between mastectomy and lumpectomy. But to make that choice, a woman needs to understand her subsequent choices. Before deciding on a lumpectomy she needs to understand the basics of radiation treatment, because breast-conserving surgery is almost always accompanied by a course of such therapy. Before deciding on a mastectomy she needs to grapple with the pros and cons of reconstructive surgery—with a number of reconstructive alternatives, such as "the transverse rectus abdominus myocutaneous flap" and "the deep inferior epigastric perforator flap."

The assortment of decisions and the information required to comprehend each option can be overwhelming. Ideally, each woman facing these decisions would meet specialists from surgery, plastics, and radiation before choosing between mastectomy and lumpectomy. But that is not how most women make their choice. Paula knew immediately, almost instinctively, that she wanted a lumpectomy, unless her surgeon told her that it wasn't a viable alternative.

In observing Paula's decision making, I was reminded of a famous study done of people considering whether to donate one of their kidneys to a loved one. The researchers were interested in how people weighed the pros and cons of donation, how they factored in the time their loved one would otherwise be expected to wait for a transplant, how well the regular transplant would function compared to the one they might donate, and whether donating a kidney would cause them, the donors, acute or chronic health problems. In other words, a cascade of trade-offs. How did people make this complicated decision? Their thought processes typically went something like this:

"Our tests show that you are a good match for your brother. So we wondered—"

"Yes!"

"—if you would be willing to—huh?"

"Yes, I'll donate."

Most people made their decision before learning anything about the risks and benefits of the procedure. Only then did they listen to the pros and cons of donation. The researchers had set out to study the process of what experts called "informed consent," whereby patients would first be informed about their alternatives before deciding whether to consent to any of them. But the kidney donors hadn't gotten the memo. They preferred doing things backward—consent followed by information.

This backward approach to kidney donation isn't that different from how many of us make decisions in our lives. We generate quick and strong impressions of our alternatives, gravitate quickly to one, and then stick by that alternative unless we receive overwhelming information favoring an alternative. That was certainly how Paula faced the choice between mastectomy and lumpectomy. In her mind, it was lumpectomy until proven otherwise. When the surgical oncologist raised questions about the cosmetic outcome of a lumpectomy, Paula looked for ways to hold on to that choice, seeking out alternatives that would improve the cosmetic outcome of a lumpectomy. Similarly, even though we hadn't met with a radiation oncologist yet, Paula asked me to find out whether radiation caused special problems for redheads. When the answer came back, through a colleague of mine, that Paula's pale skin would be no more susceptible to side effects than anyone else's, her preference for lumpectomy over mastectomy became even stronger.

Yet all the while, as she sorted through her surgical decision, Paula couldn't get her mind off another part of her potential treatment. It was time for Paula to meet with the medical oncologist to find out whether she needed chemotherapy.

RULE OF THUMB

I have already hinted at the large number of alternatives Paula had to grapple with in thinking through her surgery decision. Fortunately, Paula's oncologist quickly explained that the surgical decisions could be kept entirely separate from the chemotherapy decision. In an un-hurried manner, she explained her role on Paula's team:

"Your breast cancer team will be made up of five people. The first four are" (she held out her hand and grabbed hold of one of her fingers as she mentioned each specialty) "the surgical oncologist, the plastic surgeon, the pathologist, and the radiation oncologist. They concern themselves with your local disease, doing what they can to keep the breast cancer from returning in your left breast. Now me," she said. "I am the thumb." She pointed her thumb in our direction. "I worry about cancer in the rest of your body. My job is to keep your cancer from showing up anywhere else."

In the last thirty years medical experts have learned that breast cancer is a systemic disease. By the time breast cancer is large enough to detect by mammography, it has typically spread to distant parts of the body. In worst-case scenarios, this spread involves metastases, with new masses growing in bone, brain, or elsewhere. More often, the spread is only microscopic: somewhere in the woman's body, cancer cells have traveled with the intention of settling down, if left undisturbed for enough time. Back in the days of Betty Ford, most experts considered localized breast cancer to be just that—localized and therefore a surgical disease. Experts assumed that breast cancer spread locally and methodically. According to this assumption, if surgery fails to cure breast cancer, if a patient has metastases at a later date, then the operation must have been too timid. A more aggressive treatment, the thinking went, would have removed more cancer cells and thereby prevented recurrence.

With the failure of the radical mastectomy to benefit women, breast cancer clinicians realized that the key to long-term cancer-free survival isn't simply to remove tissue. It's to find medications—chemotherapies—that circulate through the rest of the body, destroying cancer cells that have escaped the reach of the scalpel.

Chemotherapy. The word filled Paula's mind with images of head scarves and nausea. Not one who likes to be the center of attention, Paula hoped to avoid physical signs of illness that would inevitably generate comments. She wasn't worried about being ashamed. Betty Ford's decision to make her illness public had been a huge step forward in destigmatizing breast cancer. Instead, the opposite problem loomed larger in Paula's mind. Breast cancer is so visible these days, with survivors wearing their scarves almost as a badge of courage; Paula was worried that showing visible signs of her diagnosis would result in too much "You go, girl!" sentiment. Paula didn't want to hear how "brave" or "strong" she was. She didn't want to wear pink ribbons or yellow wristbands. She just wanted to deal with her illness in private, living life as normally as possible. After all, this is a woman who, when e-mailing friends to inform them of her diagnosis, ended her message with "P.S. I hate pink."

And now we were meeting with the oncologist, who would be telling us what poisons would be best for Paula and when she would begin administering them. The oncologist looked over Paula's biopsy result and her radiology reports. She explained that even though we had important information already—we knew the size of the tumor, for example, and its estrogen receptor status—we needed a few more pieces of information before we could make a final treatment decision. "It's too early to know what treatment you'll need," she told Paula. "But if I had to guess, and I'm a good guesser, I'd say you won't need chemotherapy. We should be able to treat your cancer with endocrine therapy."

Paula's face lit up. Endocrine therapy—medications like tamoxifen and Femara—targeted the hormones in Paula's system that, if undeterred, would prompt her tumor to grow. These antihormone drugs had side effects of their own and would force Paula into early menopause, but they were much less toxic than chemotherapy. No hair loss, no scarves, no barf buckets! She was ecstatic.

But I had a different reaction. I found myself obsessing on the word "guess." This was only a guess, I told myself. Why would the oncologist get Paula's hopes up if she weren't sure what treatment she would need? Paula's emotions were rising and falling like a mountain stage in the Tour de France. The surgeon had stepped outside of his expertise to tell Paula that she probably needed chemotherapy and now the oncologist, working within her expertise, had "guessed" that Paula wouldn't need chemotherapy.

I spent the next few days managing Paula's expectations: "Yes, it's great news, babe. You might not need chemotherapy. But let's not go any further than that. For all we know, you might end up getting chemo anyway. Let's just wait for all the data to come in to prepare for whatever comes." My words had their usual effect on Paula's thinking. She took in what I had to say, and then told all her friends that she wouldn't need chemo.

NINETY-SIX GRAMS

Her worries about chemotherapy behind her for now, Paula focused on the looming surgical decision. It had been more than two weeks since her diagnosis and she was eager to get on with things. Yet not so eager that she rushed into a mastectomy. There was time, first, to talk with a plastic surgeon about the chance that she might still be a candidate for a lumpectomy.

The plastic surgeon came recommended to us as a technical wizard. When he entered the room, Paula was already sitting on the exam table, her hospital gown on backward so that the size and shape of her breasts were easier to see. The plastic surgeon palpated her tumor to assess how much tissue would need to be removed if she got a lumpectomy. "You'll definitely need reconstruction," he said. "But I can do that at the time of the surgery."

I was confused. I thought we were seeing him for advice about whether Paula could get a lumpectomy. But now he was talking like she would need a mastectomy. That choice, to my knowledge, was the only surgical option paired with immediate reconstruction. Once again, my incomplete knowledge had caused me to leap to an erroneous conclusion, because he was describing a much newer approach to breast cancer reconstruction, a procedure in the relatively new field of oncoplasty. He explained that right after the surgical oncologist removed the tumor, he could reshape Paula's breast. Or was it breasts? I couldn't tell, because he was talking so quickly.

He continued describing treatment options. One option he clearly preferred, the option of immediate bilateral breast reduction. "I would take the tissue remaining in your left breast—" He was now drawing a picture. "And rearrange it so it has a nice shape. Then I would reduce your right breast, so its size roughly matches the left."

Paula nodded along eagerly with a broad grin on her face. He knew from experience that most women Paula's age would be delighted at the idea of smaller, less gravitationally challenged breasts.

"Now, there is a downside to immediate reconstruction," he continued. "The radiation will potentially shrink your left breast. It can take up to a year for that breast to reach its final size. So if I do immediate reconstruction, when the left breast finishes shrinking, it might not perfectly match the right. I'll take that into consideration when doing the initial procedure. But I don't see that as a problem. You've already tolerated a fair amount of asymmetry," he said, looking back at Paula's still-exposed breasts. "It looks like your right breast is about ninety-six grams larger than your left, so we should stay well within that degree of asymmetry."

I don't want to get too far into too-much-information territory here, but I had by then spent a bit more time looking at and touching my wife's breasts than this guy, and I had never noticed any kind of asymmetry. The plastic surgeon not only noticed this asymmetry but had it pegged at ninety-six grams?

His explanations continued so rapidly that I couldn't dwell on his asymmetry comment. He told us that we could delay reconstruction of the left breast until after radiation, but that this option would leave the breast tissue harder to reshape. (At least I think that's what he said.) He explained that he could reconstruct the left breast immediately and hold off on reconstructing the right side until the final size of Paula's left breast was established, thereby guaranteeing a perfect match. But that would mean a year of substantial asymmetry, plus a second surgery. Paula didn't like that option at all.

He raced through another scenario or two, and I was completely lost. I tried to slow things down:

"So, if I'm hearing you right, we have four options?"

"Uh-huh."

"And I guess the first option is . . ."

He waved me off dismissively. Already behind in his schedule, he was in no mood to wait for me to slog through the list. He stated with a measure of finality, "Our best option is immediate bilateral reconstruction." He then explained how he would coordinate his procedure with that of the surgical oncologist. He talked about finding a date when their schedules were both free. And then . . .

He was gone. I was dumbfounded. I couldn't figure out how we had arrived at a decision. But Paula looked happy, really happy with what we, or they, or he had decided upon. And I sat there wondering how I could have been so passive. It would be several weeks before I understood the full consequences of my passivity.

In previous chapters I have written about several new interventions that promise to prepare patients to be active partners in their medical decisions: decision aids that inform people of their treatment alternatives, DVDs that teach them how to interact with their physicians, even decision coaches to help patients talk in a language that their physicians understand. Yet when we left the plastic surgeon's office that day I didn't feel as if we had actively partnered in the decision. Instead, I felt shut out. Intimidated, actually. I had tried to ask questions, using the very techniques I had built into my prostate cancer DVD, and I had been dismissed with a wave of his busy hand. I'm embarrassed to say that I even felt a bit guilty for asking too many questions.

The activated patient is no match for an indifferent clinician. Even Paula was unusually uncritical about the decisions we were making. This from a woman who is famous for her relentlessness.

Take, for instance, her reaction to a seven-cent bill from our cable television company. One year, Paula's mother underpaid the cable company by seven cents when closing down their family's cabin. Paula thought it was ridiculous to waste a stamp and an envelope to pay the bill, as well as waste the time of some employee at the cable company whose job it was to process the payment. So she went to the cable company website to pay electronically only to find that the company required a one-dollar minimum payment. She called a "billing specialist" and explained the situation. The—ahem—specialist, clearly reading off a script, stated, "I'm sorry but the balance is a legitimate charge so we cannot waive the fee." To which Paula replied, "I understand that, but it would be cheaper to ignore the seven cents."

"I'm sorry but the balance is a legitimate charge so . . ."

Paula began giving her credit card information to the specialist but was quickly cut off. "I'm sorry, ma'am, but we would have to charge you two dollars for paying over the phone by credit card." This really got Paula going now. She was trying to be nice and save them time and money. So she went onto her bank website, which she thought would be able to send an e-check to the company at no cost (and without killing trees). But she was thwarted again—it too required a one-dollar minimum payment.

Most people would have given up long before this point, but Paula wasn't finished. She had one last trick up her sleeve. She sent the e-check to the cable company at the aforementioned one-dollar-minimum value. Two weeks later, she contacted the cable company and asked them to send *her* a check for the credit balance of ninety-three cents that was now in the account.

What I am trying to paint here is a picture of a highly empowered, unintimidated, and wickedly clever woman who I never would have guessed would leave that plastic surgeon's office with a treatment plan lined up even though neither of us understood the alternatives as well as we should have. Paula was now scheduled for a lumpectomy with bilateral reconstruction. We mistakenly thought our first major decision was behind us.

A SENTINEL MOMENT

During the several weeks between Paula's diagnosis and her surgery, word spread through the medical community of a landmark trial proving that breast cancer surgery no longer needed to be as invasive as it had become. The new trial tested the value of axillary lymph node dissection in women with operable breast cancer. Half of the women in the trial underwent the current standard of care: They received either a lumpectomy or a mastectomy plus a biopsy of their sentinel lymph nodes. Sentinel nodes stand as an early warning sign that a tumor has established itself outside the breast. Under this standard of care, if one of these sentinel nodes reveals metastasis, the surgeon removes the remaining nodes. This standard is based on the assumption that the more local tissue the surgeon removes, the less tumor remains for other treatments, like chemotherapy, to kill.

Putting that assumption to the test, the other half of the women in this study were not given any further lymph node surgery, even if one of their sentinel nodes contained cancer. The theory underlying this approach was that systemic therapies like chemotherapy would knock off any cancer cells in those lymph nodes. The study confirmed this alternative theory to be correct. A full fifteen years after the surgery, there was no difference in survival rate between these two groups of women. The surgical standard of care was deemed unnecessarily aggressive.

I was ecstatic. Paula would not need to have her lymph nodes removed. Even better, she would be less likely to experience what many women find to be the worst side effect of breast cancer surgery, lymphedema. Women with breast cancer often experience chronic arm swelling as a result of receiving lymph node dissection. The swelling can be triggered by exercise or a long airplane flight. Once triggered, the swelling can become permanent. To combat this often-painful condition, women are forced to wear long compression sleeves, making their affected arms feel like Civil War belles in size-zero corsets.

When I gave Paula a kiss on the morning of her surgery and watched the nurses roll her toward the operating room, I was content in the knowledge that she would be receiving the newest, most minimalist breast cancer surgery in the history of modern medicine. You can now understand my shock when the surgeon tracked me down in the middle of the operation to ask me whether I wanted him to "remove more lymph nodes." I couldn't see how this was necessary anymore.

"What do you think Paula would want?" he asked.

"Well, . . . I don't know. I mean, didn't that recent study show that . . ."

"Ah, the *New England Journal* study. You saw that. Yes, I was involved in that research. I have looked closely at the data."

"Uh-huh."

"And it turns out that Paula's cancer is more advanced than most of the patients in that study."

"More advanced?"

"Yes. In that study the lymph node metastases were not identified in the frozen sections but were only visible in the permanent sections. Most of the metastases in that study were quite small. I am sorry to tell you that Paula's metastasis was a full centimeter in size, easily identifiable in frozen section."

My mind was racing now. My best friend, my life partner, had a metastasis. A big one too. I had clearly been kidding myself that her cancer would be a harmless lesion, a temporary nuisance. I sat there shocked that it had already spread into her armpit. But I couldn't take any time to sort through my shock, because I had to decide whether to let this surgeon remove more of Paula's lymph nodes, exposing her to the risk of lymphedema. And for what? The hypothetical chance that these additional excisions would prolong her life? Would slow down her tumor?

I pushed back. "But there's no evidence that the dissection would help her, is there?"

"Well, no. We haven't done a randomized trial in people like Paula. But her metastasis . . . it's not something I could easily ignore. I'd feel better going in and removing more nodes. But what's really important is figuring out what Paula would want. Would she want to talk this through with me before undergoing any more surgery?"

Of course she would love to talk to you, I thought. Hell, she would have really loved to talk to you *before* the surgery. Why are we having this conversation now? My brain raced as I tried to figure out what Paula would want. I knew she despised surgery. I knew that anesthesia makes her sick and that her recovery is almost always more painful than average. Redheads, she had often reminded me, are more sensitive to pain than other people.

But Paula would despise lymphedema too. And why the heck is this surgeon so confident in the value of further dissection? Of all the husbands to be having this conversation, why did it have to be me, a man so steeped in information about the history of breast cancer treatment?

My clinical instincts told me that further surgery would be unnecessary, that in time we'd all look back and wonder why we went after lymph nodes so aggressively. But I also thought of Paula lying on the table, and of the likelihood that when she woke up the surgeon would convince her to undergo the lymph node dissection, and of her undergoing another operation, and . . . and I told him to go ahead and remove more lymph nodes.

"Okay, I'll take as few as I can," he replied.

I wish I could say that we were done with surprises.

YOU LOOK RADIANT

After Paula returned home from surgery and had begun recovery from the procedure, I told her about my conversation with the surgeon. I dreaded the thought that I had let her down, but she assured me that I had made the right decision. I suspect she was trying to keep me from feeling guilty. What a sweetheart!

Her wounds healed nicely over the next couple of weeks, meaning she could begin radiation treatment. Lumpectomy, you may remember, only works as well as mastectomy when accompanied by radiation.

Radiation treatment has come a long way since the days when zealous practitioners aimed high doses of cobalt at unsuspecting patients like Irma Natanson, whom we met in chapter 1. Now radiation oncologists aim their beams with almost molecular precision, thereby limiting the amount of collateral damage experienced by surrounding tissue. The radiation oncology resident explained these facts to us in elaborate yet not overwhelming detail, giving us a minitutorial that not only informed us of what they were planning to do but also calmed many of our fears about the hazards of this otherwise barbaric-sounding treatment. We were told to expect six weeks of therapy, with the main side effects being fatigue and a mild sunburn-like reaction.

Then the senior radiation oncologist came into the room and re-explained many of these same facts to us. She was another great explainer, a physician clearly dedicated to good communication. She confirmed a number of the details of Paula's medical history as she reviewed the chart. She examined Paula's surgical wounds, to see if they had healed sufficiently enough to weather the storm of radiation soon coming their way.

"Looks great. We should be able to start next week."

"Great," said Paula.

"As Sherri [the resident] explained to you already, we will start with five weeks of treatment to the entire breast. We'll also include your axilla because of the positive lymph node."

"Yep."

"Now, we normally would have followed that up with a sixth week of treatment, what we call a boost to the tumor bed. We would have focused a beam onto the area where your tumor used to be, to reduce the chance of the cancer returning there. But because you have already had reconstructive surgery, and the plastic surgeon rearranged your remaining breast tissue, we no longer know exactly where your tumor bed lies. So we'll just stick with the five weeks of treatment. That means that next Thursday we can schedule you for . . ."

She delivered this news with a reassuring smile on her face and without a hint of disappointment, but I sat in stunned silence. How had we given the green light to immediate reconstructive surgery without knowing that this would impact Paula's radiation treatment? Once again, we had failed to think through an important decision because the pace of medical progress had outrun our knowledge. No, wait. That's not fair. The problem wasn't that we failed to think. We didn't even know there was a decision to think about! Paula's oncoplastic procedure was still relatively new, an advance that hadn't made it into the decision aid or into my general awareness as a physician. The plastic surgeon should have told us about this issue. Or someone on the health-care team should have made sure we had spoken with the radiation oncologist *before* the surgery, so Paula could have decided whether this oncoplastic procedure was so much better than the alternatives that she'd be willing to forgo the sixth week of boost therapy. But no one—not either of the surgeons or the oncologist—seemed to be aware that this would be an issue. And now, as a result, Paula would have to be content with a five-week course of radiation treatment. Astonishing. Truly astonishing.

The radiation oncologist continued telling us more details about Paula's treatment, patiently and clearly answering each of our questions. Then we drove home, both of us putting the boost controversy out of our minds. No reason to dwell on things beyond our control.

A couple of days later, Paula and I sent an e-mail to our friends, updating them on Paula's progress and on her remaining treatment. I quickly received a response (not copied to Paula) from my radiation oncology friend, the one who had let us know earlier that redheads don't have unique problems tolerating such treatments. She was surprised. "You know," she wrote, "six weeks would be standard treatment. Aren't they planning to do a boost?" I e-mailed back explaining the situation, and she quickly backpedaled: "Well, the boost brings only limited benefits. Nothing to worry about."

But I wasn't in a mood to be told what qualified as something to be worried about. So I asked my friend to send me articles about boost treatment. She e-mailed me a report on a large randomized trial, the study that had established boost therapy as the standard of care. I'll cut to the chase. In the subset of women who most closely resembled Paula, clinically speaking, the boost reduced localized breast cancer recurrence by 8 percent over fifteen years, from around 15 percent to 7 percent. That is a pretty substantial reduction in recurrence. But reduction at a cost, because as I dug deeper into the article, I saw that the boost also increases the odds of experiencing moderate or severe breast fibrosis. Think of breast fibrosis as scar tissue deep in the breast that causes the breast to pucker or feel hard. Fibrosis can affect the breast's appearance, distorting its shape. In addition, it can alter breast sensation. An area of fibrosis can tighten into an almost mass-like state, causing some women to mistakenly conclude that they have experienced cancer recurrences. Extrapolating data from the study, I calculated that Paula's chance of breast fibrosis would rise from 10 percent to 30 percent if she received the boost.

What the radiation oncologist saw as the standard of care looked very much to me like a preference-sensitive decision, the kind of trade-off where it would be hard to find fault with a woman who chose to forgo the boost.

Now I found myself truly confused. Should I be upset because we weren't given the chance by our surgeon to have the boost? Or would that chance have been moot, since the radiation oncologist wouldn't have given us a choice anyway? It was clear to me that if Paula had had a more traditional lumpectomy, we would have been told that she needed six weeks of therapy, and I never would have known that the sixth week of boost therapy was optional and depended on Paula's preferences.

The only reason I was able to recognize the boost decision as a trade-off was because I read the original study (and because I am, as you know by now, obsessed with preference-sensitive decisions).

THE NEED TO PREPARE DOCTORS FOR PREPARED PATIENTS

Over the next couple of months Paula made her way through the medical system in strong shape. She flew through her radiation treatment without any acute complications. She was able to get the sixth week of treatment too—the boost—in part because I put our radiation oncologist in touch with a friend of mine, a well-known radiation oncologist who explained why that treatment was still feasible. The best news came when radiation was complete. We found out that Paula didn't need chemotherapy. One bullet dodged and, consequently, one very happy wife. A wife who soon had energy again to attend to her job and, of course, to look closely at things like our monthly cable bill.

But our trip through the world of breast cancer treatment had been far too bumpy. Our experience had revealed the limits of patient empowerment.

The idea that informed patients would be able to make medical decisions was always naïve. Most patients aren't ready to assert themselves in the context of a medical exam room, much less when lying sick in a hospital bed. Even efforts to "activate" patients—with interventions like DVDs designed to prepare patients for their doctor visit or decision coaches willing to come along to each appointment—seem inadequate in the face of a health-care system populated by physicians who don't know how to share the decision-making burden. It is hard for empowered patients to participate in decisions when medical information moves more quickly than they can absorb it. It is hard for activated patients to ask questions of busy clinicians who know how to exit an exam room on time. It is impossible to insert patient preferences into preference-sensitive decisions when the doctors don't even recognize the nature of the trade-off and believe incorrectly that one size—the standard of care—fits all.

I believe in empowering patients but not in order to make them into solo decision makers. In most circumstances, the real reason to empower patients is so that they can partner with their health-care team in making decisions. The patient-empowerment revolution is being transformed into a shared decision-making movement. But for patients to be able to partner in their decisions, they need to encounter doctors who are prepared to interact with prepared patients. In other words, we need to teach physicians how to share.

THIRTEEN

Preparing Physicians
for Prepared Patients

Roger Robinson inserted the CD-ROM into his computer and began listening to the same conversation he had participated in only a short while ago, another doctor–patient encounter gone bad. The patient, who was suffering from metastatic cancer, had pleaded for understanding from his doctor. But the oncologist was oblivious to his concerns.

As we've already seen, too often patients come into their doctors' offices unprepared for the encounter—unschooled in how to communicate within the constraints of the typical fifteen-minute appointment and unfamiliar with the language and culture of physician–patient interactions. But we've also seen how interventions—like CD-ROMs, DVDs, and websites—can better prepare patients for these encounters, turning the unfamiliar into something more predictable.

But Roger Robinson wasn't reviewing this encounter to familiarize himself with the normal ways in which doctors and patients interact. Nor was he doing so to acquaint himself with the particular jargon he could expect to hear during subsequent conversations. Indeed, if anyone was contributing jargon to this conversation, it was Robinson, because Robinson wasn't the patient in this conversation. He was the oncologist.

Robinson was participating in a study led by James Tulsky, a physician at Duke University who was conducting an experiment to figure out what would happen if doctors were given a chance to listen to themselves. I will tell you more about Tulsky's study later and the dramatic effect it had on how doctors like Robinson behaved during subsequent patient encounters, but I bring up Tulsky's study in order to give you a preview of how we can transform medical decisions into shared affairs.

In the beginning, as we have seen, the patient-empowerment revolution was about power. Leaders of the revolution believed that doctors had held too much power for too long. They concluded that doctors needed to be stripped of some of their power. Hence, they waged battle with physicians in court, harnessing the power of the law to force physicians to abandon their paternalistic ways. They also skirmished with the establishment in the pages of the leading medical journals, with ethicists arguing that patients had rights and that doctors had the duty to respect those rights. They even developed interventions that would empower patients. The ends of the revolution would be achieved, they believed, through informed-consent documents and interactive decision aids.

But a revolution only succeeds if the two sides settle at some point upon a new balance of power. The patient-empowerment revolution needs to step aside for a better alternative, a shared decision-making movement. To reach this goal, we can't simply inform and activate patients. We also need to re-educate doctors. The biggest challenge to shared decision making today is not a lack of patient empowerment. As much as we need to increase our efforts to inform patients about their treatment alternatives and to teach them how to be active partners in their decisions, these efforts won't lead to good decision making unless patients are paired off with enlightened physicians. Jack Wennberg and his colleagues came up with the idea of decision aids in part because they were at loggerheads with Bob Brook and other people at RAND who were convinced that the way to improve decision making was to re-educate physicians. Wennberg thought patients needed information; Brook thought doctors needed more guidance. In retrospect, both groups were right. The success of the shared decision-making revolution depends on both ends of the stethoscope.

As we saw in chapter 9, when Mary Smith came to Dartmouth for breast cancer care, she almost gave in to her surgeon's preference for a mastectomy because she wanted to be a good patient. Even after reviewing a breast cancer decision aid, she wasn't confident enough about her own preferences, and her own role in the decision, to push back. It was only after she had met with her plastic surgeon—E. Dale Collins Vidal, a leader in the shared decision-making movement—that she gathered the courage to ask for a lumpectomy. The decision aid wasn't enough to empower her to make her own choice or even, for that matter, to convince her to discuss her preferences with the surgeon.

When my wife, Paula, was diagnosed with breast cancer, we were lucky to receive medical care from a group of generous and kind physicians. But we were not fortunate enough to work with doctors who truly understood shared decision making. We partnered with a surgical oncologist who didn't think to discuss lymph node dissection until halfway through Paula's operation. We collaborated with a plastic surgeon who didn't find it necessary to tell us that his reconstructive technique might interfere with the radiation treatment. And we teamed up with a radiation specialist who didn't believe that the choice of whether to receive a sixth week of radiation was . . . a choice! Despite the sincere gratitude that I have for the excellent care each of these physicians provided to my wife, I don't feel as if any of our interactions achieved the ideals of partnership. None were true collaborations.

To achieve the goals of the shared decision-making revolution, we not only need to educate and activate patients, we also need to prepare physicians to interact with prepared patients. We need to retrain physicians like Roger Robinson in the basic art of communication. We need to modernize medical education to take advantage of advances in the behavioral and decision sciences, which point toward better methods of making decisions with patients. And we need to think long and hard about the best ways to select people for the medical profession who have an aptitude for handling the challenging world of medical decision making.

INTERVIEW DAY

They stood in the hallway, adorned in gray suits, their futures as physicians hanging in the balance. It was medical school interview day, and the hopeful applicants were participating in an exercise that resembled speed dating with Socrates. No hour-long interviews with esteemed faculty. Instead, the applicants raced through a series of two-minute interviews during which they discussed difficult medical dilemmas with medical school faculty. In the first round of interviews, Student No. 1 was asked to discuss the pros and cons of requiring patients to pay out of pocket for expensive medical tests; Student No. 2 was asked to discuss whether it is wrong for doctors to give unproven treatments to their patients; Students No. 3 through 12 tackled alternative dilemmas. Then, the bell rang and the students rotated places. One interview down, eleven to go.

When I applied to medical school in the early 1980s, most schools set me up with two or three hour-long interviews. "Why do you want to be a doctor?" they'd ask, a question which it was safe to say most students were prepared to answer. At most schools, interviewers also asked me about my unusual undergraduate background. "I see you studied philosophy and music," one interviewer said to me. "They always ask me to interview the humanities majors," he continued, "because I'm the only English major on the admissions committee." These lengthy interviews were time consuming for applicants and for medical school faculty, time essentially wasted if the school was hoping to use the interviews to determine which applicants were best suited to becoming physicians, because most research suggests that these interviews do nothing to predict success in medical school or beyond. They certainly don't predict later performance in clinical settings, when students are assessed for things like communication skills. In fact, absent some kind of sociopathic behavior, interviews often have little impact on whether students are accepted into medical school, acceptance or rejection typically based instead on numbers like GPA and test scores.

Grades and test scores in science and math have been the key to becoming a doctor since at least the 1950s. After all, physicians are applied scientists (or at least that's the conventional wisdom) who use science to heal people. Moreover, many physicians use their knowledge of science to develop new ways of healing patients. (The Nobel Prize in Medicine could just as easily be called the Nobel Prize in Applied Biological Sciences.) With such a strong emphasis on scientific knowledge, it is easier for a math whiz with Asperger's to get into a medical school than a calculus-challenged art history major with an astronomical social IQ.

The goal of those speed-dating interviews—officially known as the multiple mini-interview—is to identify applicants who are more than just organic chemistry stars. The existence of these mini-interviews at a handful of schools is a sign of recognition among leaders of the profession that things aren't right in the trenches. The profession's emphasis on scientific and technical wizardry has led medical schools to admit too many of the wrong students, people who have been conditioned by their science training to look for black-and-white solutions—sodium plus chloride equals table salt; the square root of thirty-six does not equal nine. The world of medical diagnosis and treatment is often far messier than a chemistry lab, with black and white replaced by a kaleidoscope of grays. In clinical settings, doctors often can't be sure of their patients' diagnoses. Even when a diagnosis is obvious, the best course of treatment may not be apparent. Add in the messiness of patient preferences, with one patient favoring one thing and another favoring an alternative, and many of these former biochemistry stars struggle. Memorizing chemical pathways didn't prepare them for this!

The mini-interviews are designed to better identify people who are constitutionally suited to practice medicine. Thus, interviewers ask applicants to discuss ethical dilemmas that don't have straightforward right or wrong answers so that the schools can assess the applicant's ability to remain open-minded and deal with uncertainty. The interviews also aim to pick up on people skills that might not be crucial in getting good grades in physics. "We are trying to weed out the students who look great on paper but haven't developed the people or communication skills we think are important," says Dr. Stephen Workman, the associate dean for admissions and administration at Virginia Tech Carilion, one of the schools that makes prominent use of this interview technique.

Early evidence suggests that the mini-interview procedure is better than the old interview procedure. For instance, students who perform well in the mini-interview also tend to perform well in medical school when participating in "structured clinical encounters," interactions with patients that are set up so that teachers can observe students' communication skills and problem-solving abilities. With the help of interventions like the multiple mini-interview, there is hope that the next generation of doctors will be better suited to the complex decisions that make up much of medical care.

But even this change will not bring a quick end to many of the decision-making foibles I have described in this book. For starters, it will take twenty or thirty years to repopulate the profession with these new and improved physicians. Moreover, the communication and decision-making problems I've written about are the result of many social and psychological forces that won't go away, even if we succeed in enrolling more diverse and socially skilled students into the medical profession. Take the jargon problem I discussed in chapter 3. Students don't enter medical schools believing that the best way to tell a patient he has leukemia is to say that "your peripheral smear showed immature cells." Even students chosen by traditional means, who've spent their college years with their noses buried in biology textbooks, are not so clueless as to think that physicians should follow up on sentences like "you have cancer" with paragraphs of arcane details on the histopathology of the patient's tumor. The often-inscrutable ways in which doctors talk to their patients is not simply a product of who gets accepted to medical school. It's also a consequence of the way we train students once they enter medical school. It's nurture over nature.

If we truly want to improve physician communication and bring new doctors into the profession who are ready and willing to work with activated patients, we need to pay attention not only to *who* we educate as physicians but also *how* we educate them.

GENETIC DETERMINISM

The faculty at the University of Pennsylvania called him "neutron Bill" because, as CEO of the hospital and dean of the medical school, he didn't hesitate to get rid of anyone who failed to meet his standards. After he arrived in the early 1990s, the buildings survived but not necessarily the people, as if the medical center had been hit by a neutron bomb. Bill Kelley was a world-famous physician widely admired for his medical knowledge, universally revered for his groundbreaking research, and genuinely feared due to the expectations he had of his employees. "I only ask my faculty to work half-time," he reportedly said. "What they do the other twelve hours each day of the week is none of my business." Before coming to Penn, Kelley had been chairman of internal medicine at the University of Michigan, a post he took at the astonishingly young age of thirty-six. (This is a position most people don't attain until well into their fifties.) He had built the department at Michigan into one of the world's strongest, and now he planned to take an already strong medical school at Penn and move it up to "number one in NIH funding," as he used to say. And he planned to do so by focusing on genes.

In a faculty meeting early in Kelley's tenure, he explained with characteristic confidence that patients' genes are the roots of all illness; thus, the key to curing patients is to understand (and even modify) their genes. It was a bravura performance. He energized the audience with his ambitious vision. But this being a faculty audience, there were inevitably a few gadflies in the room. One skeptical faculty member asked how infections could be blamed on human genes. Kelley shot back that not all humans are equally susceptible to infectious organisms, so we needed to focus on what genes reside in resistant humans.

I shared this person's skepticism. But as a new faculty member, and one who was quite far away from receiving tenure, I kept my mouth shut. This wasn't the right time or place to question the over-molecularization of illness. Nevertheless, I felt astonished by this incredibly reductionist view of illness. What about smoking? Was the problem simply that some humans lack the genes that would make them resistant to the unhealthy consequences of tobacco? What about obesity? Should we stop counseling our patients about diet and exercise and focus our efforts instead on identifying genes that keep us thin, even when we lie around eating potato chips?

I remember Kelley's talk because, as a new faculty member, it brought back painful memories of my first two years of medical school, when I was forced to memorize anatomical nomenclature that had never once helped me care for a sick patient. It was the Kelleys of the world, I told myself, who had subjected me to all that useless minutiae, all the while providing me with only scant instruction in topics more relevant to medical care. I was given a few days of instruction on how to talk to patients, but even that content was centered on "how to take a medical history"—how to ask questions, in other words, that would help me diagnose my patients' illnesses, not how to best discern my patients' emotional states or to assess whether patients understood what I was telling them. In my first two years of medical school—the didactic years, when I attended lecture classes—I received an hour or two of instruction on doctor–patient communication, a single practice session with a standardized patient (an actor hired to pose as a patient), and a few ethics lectures about the importance of involving patients in their health-care decisions. But the lecturers didn't describe any techniques on how to do this. It was all theory and no practical wisdom.

The rest of my training—the last two years of medical school and the duration of my residency—took place mainly in clinical settings. The clean and organized world of lectures and tests was distant history. I was now immersed in the real world, tackling problems as they chaotically unfolded. It is during these clinical years that most students develop the bedside manner they will carry forward through their careers, forming habits that will influence the way they talk to patients about preference-sensitive decisions. Sadly, they too often develop these patterns and habits with insufficient feedback and scant structural guidance. During my clinical training, I learned by observing senior physicians when they spoke with patients, but usually these interactions were brief and unaccompanied by didactic reflection. I don't remember many senior physicians pulling me aside and explaining why they had framed a decision one way to a patient rather than another way. It was up to me to figure out what made some of my mentors better communicators than others. Bedside manner was part of the "art of medicine," we were told. Consequently, it was not seen as a rigorous skill that could be developed through careful instruction or as a practice that could be informed by science. Contrast that with the physical exam—I can't count how many times I was shown how to examine a patient's abdomen or how often I was given a quick lecture on how to interpret specific skin findings.

Admittedly, I completed medical school and residency in the late 1980s. Instruction has changed since then. Many of the schools I have lectured at in recent years have beefed up their instruction on topics like communication. But usually this training is provided during medical school and drifts by the wayside during residency. For example, I recently spent several mornings observing hospital teams at a leading university. In a span of over three hours, the team I observed spent only ten minutes at the bedside of their patient. They spent the remaining time in a conference room, where various members of the medical team scrolled through computer screens, pulling up lab data and X-ray reports. The team had lots of data to pore over that morning and lots of clinical facts to discuss, but ten minutes? How can new doctors develop skill at the bedside if their teachers don't spend time at the bedside with them?

Not only do students and residents get very little chance to watch experienced clinicians interview patients, they often get even less opportunity to be observed by experienced clinicians while they interview a patient. In my entire residency, I can't recall *ever* being observed while I conducted an interview of a patient, or being taught how to have difficult conversations with patients, or how to give them bad news. I don't remember being evaluated by my superiors on how I handled such situations. This lack of observation and guidance contrasts sharply with the way we teach other aspects of medical practice. No surgeon completes training without being observed hundreds of times in the operating room, until senior surgeons are convinced that she has good operative technique. No internist finishes residency without being quizzed scores of times about their interpretation of patients' electrolyte disturbances or EKG readings. But both observation and lessons on helping patients make decisions that reflect their preferences are essentially absent from clinical training. There are notable exceptions to this absence, clinicians who emphasize the bedside in their teaching and who convey communication skills to their students, not just diagnostic techniques. In addition, some medical schools and residencies place much more emphasis on the softer side of medicine than others. But the dominant model of medical training is still one that gives huge priority to pathophysiology over psychology, and to the biological determinants of illness over the social ones.

Part of the problem lies in the molecular view of illness that dominates medical school faculty, the "genes determine everything" mind-set. Most medical school deans and department chairs made their reputations running basic biology or chemistry labs, where they uncovered molecular clues that would help determine the cause, or the cure, for various diseases. They built huge research labs with NIH grants, the NIH itself being an organization dominated by basic biological scientists. This emphasis on molecules and DNA has had a tremendous impact on physicians' abilities to treat a whole array of illness.

The very drugs now circulating through my wife's system to treat her breast cancer are the result of those twelve-hour-a-day physician scientists. I'm grateful that so many brilliant, hardworking physicians have found the time to run back and forth between their patients and their research labs. But I'm also disturbed that the dominance of molecular biology in academic hospitals has created an overly reductionist view of medical education. Most medical leaders believe, first and foremost, that medical students and residents should be grounded in science. I'm reminded of a conversation a friend of mine had with his medical school dean. My friend, who is an expert in palliative care and doctor–patient communication, explained that he was researching "conversations about death and dying." The dean got all excited. "End-of-life care?" he said. "We have something in common. I am interested in cell death!" Imagine trying to interest that dean in adding a new course in how to break bad news to patients.

To achieve a goal of shared decision making, we need to change the way we train medical students and residents, with less emphasis on how molecules work and more on how humans behave. This change won't come easily. It is hard to convince a man who has committed his adult life to cell death, who has achieved success by spending his weekends and evenings with pipettes and centrifuges, that he needs to add more social scientists to his faculty or that he needs to jettison a few dozen lectures on topics like cytoplasmic mitochondria in order to teach students about body-language recognition and decision psychology.

OVERCOMING THE BARRIERS

I expect most laypeople—especially anyone who has had a bad experience interacting with a physician—don't see a problem with my suggestion of teaching doctors more about communication and decision making. But my ideas are not popular in many academic medical centers. When I have made these suggestions in front of medical school audiences, there is inevitably a rush to the microphones by physicians eager to point out my naïveté.

I have listened to each one of these physicians and fully recognize that my ideas face an uphill battle. But I believe the battle can be won. So I'm going to lay out the concerns and criticisms that I've encountered over the years and explain why none stands in the way of making the changes that will promote the shared decision-making paradigm. For those readers who practice medicine, especially those of you who work in academic medical centers, I hope the rest of this chapter will inspire you to change the way you practice medicine and improve the way you train the next generation of physicians. For everyone else, consider the rest of the chapter as a chance to peek into the ivory tower, to see the kinds of debates that are ultimately shaping the health-care system that you count on in times of need.

NO TIME TO SAY HELLO, GOOD-BYE!

When I make the case for behavioral science education to medical school audiences, I face almost universal resistance. The resistance starts around the level of people's brain stems. "We don't have room in the curriculum for new content," they will say. "We already have a hard time getting through the traditional curriculum."

I used to counter this very reasonable concern by being too contrarian for my own good. "Maybe we need to trash the traditional curriculum," I'd say.

Even those audience members who agreed with me, who felt that much of the traditional curriculum was misguided, would recoil at this suggestion: "If our schools made these changes, our students' test scores would suffer and they'd have a hard time getting into good residencies."

By suggesting such radical change, I risked taking on too many battles at once. By arguing that residency programs should care less about test scores or by suggesting that we change the board tests to reflect a wider range of skills, I was essentially asking these medical schools to shoot themselves in the foot by bucking the whole system.

I appreciate how crowded the medical school curriculum is. But now, when medical audiences complain to me about the impossibility of adding behavioral science content to the medical school curriculum, I tell them about Duke University. Duke fits the first two years of classroom didactics into fourteen months. The dean's office at Duke figured out that basic science doesn't have to take up two years of medical training. Duke students finish the traditional classroom training with ten months to spare, and there is little evidence that they or their patients suffer in response. Now, I understand that Duke's medical school is not an average school. Its students enter with higher GPAs and better test scores than most schools. But if more top schools like Duke changed their curriculum, other schools would follow. And with leadership from elite schools like Duke, board examiners will change their ways too. Duke has proven that medical students don't need two full years of basic science lectures. Questions about whether there is room in the medical curriculum for more training in behavioral science have been answered.

But an important question remains. What will it take to convince medical educators that such training deserves to become a priority? Consider Duke, again. The school made the effort to curtail the basic science curriculum not so that its students could spend those ten available months studying psychology or communication or decision making. It compressed the course work so that its students could spend ten months doing research. The problem then is not that there is no room in medical school training for more decision-relevant social sciences. The problem is that medical leaders don't want to make time for such soft science.

NO TIME FOR "SOFT SCIENCE"

Victor Strecher is a professor of public health at the University of Michigan and one of the world's leading experts in developing interventions to improve people's health behaviors. In his illustrious career, Strecher (pronounced "Streck-er") has developed interventions that help people quit smoking, persuade people to eat healthy food, remind women when it's time for a mammogram, and even convince people to exercise more regularly. His interventions have been so successful that he spun them off into a company, HealthMedia, which was bought by Johnson & Johnson in 2008 to become that company's flagship enterprise in wellness and preventive health. Strecher remains as "chief visionary" for the initiative.

In short, Strecher is a brilliant scientist. But that doesn't necessarily mean that NIH scientists were impressed by his work. Around 2008, he was invited to NIH to help its leaders get a better understanding of his research so that they could decide whether to direct more funding to behavioral science efforts. The audience, made up primarily of laboratory-based scientists, sat down to listen to Strecher with their minds open but nevertheless skeptical that they would find much value in his behavioral interventions.

Strecher started by showing the audience the design of an intervention he'd created to help people quit smoking. In his intervention, Strecher began by asking smokers a series of questions and entering their answers into a computer program that would spit out individualized interventions, tailored to the facts Strecher had learned about each smoker. Some of Strecher's tailored data were based on theories of behavior change. What stage of change, for instance, was a smoker in? Ready to quit or just beginning to think about it? Other aspects of his intervention were surprisingly mundane—repeating the smoker's name, for example, as part of the message. Strecher inserted these more mundane-sounding tailorings into his intervention in order to make the message feel more personal.

At this point in Strecher's presentation I expect most of the NIH crowd were well entertained—Strecher is a master of engaging presentations—but probably not very impressed. Theories of health behavior don't pass muster with the molecular biology crowd, who may encounter a new, common-sense-sounding theory every time they are subjected to a behavioral science lecture. (Even behavioral scientists kid themselves about the proliferation of theories in their disciplines, quipping that a theory is like a toothbrush—everyone wants one of their own, and no one wants to borrow anyone else's!) But Strecher wasn't finished. Next, he showed the NIH scientists how he'd randomized smokers to receive either a standard smoking-cessation intervention or his new, highly personalized one. He presented beautiful graphs documenting that the latter group were significantly more likely to quit smoking. I hope that at this point the audience was impressed. After all, Strecher's intervention was saving more lives than most molecules any of those scientists would develop. Even so, Strecher's intervention probably still looked, to most of the audience, like nothing more than a nice little social science experiment.

Then Strecher presented a final bit of data. He explained how he had laid a handful of smokers into an fMRI scanner, a multimillion-dollar machine designed to collect moment-by-moment information on brain activity. He had exposed them to the standard antismoking intervention and then to his tailored intervention while they lay in the scanner. And just as he had predicted, specific areas of their brain "lit up," areas known by neuroscientists to correspond with personalization, with people focusing on themselves.

The room was now abuzz. This social scientist had presented some *real* science! A Nobel laureate even rushed up to Strecher after the talk to tell him he'd never before been impressed by a behavioral science presentation.

Rationally speaking, of course, the audience should have been more impressed with Strecher's clinical results (less smoking!) than with his fMRI findings. But such is the mind-set of the biological scientist, and such is human nature, that people often have difficulty finding value in the work of those who labor in different intellectual paradigms. Social scientists, whose theories are mapped with boxes and arrows, speak a language so different from that of molecular biologists that they can't help but leave the molecular biologists unimpressed.

Now that researchers in the behavioral sciences have begun to adapt techniques and approaches to those of biologists, there is hope for behavioral science to gain some street cred. In fact, many of the phenomena I've discussed in this book have been studied in fMRI scanners. The decision psychology that informs my research has been embraced by neuroscientists who have identified which brain regions are responsible for well-known decisional biases. The field of decision psychology has also spawned new scientific disciplines, such as neuro-economics. It has even informed thinking about evolutionary biology.

In short, the gap between the social sciences and the basic biological sciences is shrinking rapidly. We are approaching a kind of "consilience," as E. O. Wilson famously called it—a unity of knowledge across disciplines. This consilience could be what we need to convince molecularly minded medical leaders to enhance their behavioral science curricula.

The time is right for medical educators to more fully embrace the behavioral sciences. There is more value in understanding human nature than in mastering the Krebs cycle.

TEACHING OLD DOGS

"It's fine to talk about changing medical school and residency education. But how will you do that when most of the faculty, the people doing the teaching, are set in their ways? How will you teach the new dogs new tricks when the old dogs only know how to roll over and play dead?"

I've been asked versions of this question a number of times by insightful audience members, and until recently I didn't have any great answers. Then came physicians like Roger Robinson, the oncologist we met at the beginning of this chapter who inserted that CD-ROM into his computer in order to listen to himself interact with one of his patients. Robinson was participating in a study led by James Tulsky, a Duke physician and researcher, a study that provides a nice example of how feasible it is to teach these old dogs some new tricks. We met Tulsky in chapter 4, when I wrote about the frequency with which physicians fail to respond to expressions of negative emotion from their patients. When Tulsky and his colleagues first discovered the dismal rates of emotional sensitivity displayed by practicing physicians, they eagerly set about advertising their findings, writing articles for leading medical journals and drafting press releases, so that word would spread. If doctors realize this problem exists, they thought, maybe they will start paying more attention to their patients' emotions. But Tulsky and his colleagues knew that publicity alone would not make these communication problems go away. They understood that doctors needed help recognizing their failures and addressing them. "We were convinced that the physicians in our studies wanted to respond appropriately to their patients' emotions. But they didn't know how to do a better job."

So Tulsky and his collaborators developed a CD-ROM that would demonstrate good communication techniques to physicians using video clips of doctor–patient encounters. Even better, before giving them the CD-ROM he also tape-recorded each physician and spliced in bits and pieces of their own encounters to illustrate places in their previous interactions where they could have improved their communication.

Tulsky took on some of the most difficult discussions physicians have with their patients. He intervened in interactions between oncologists and their sickest patients, people with stage 4 cancer. (In cancer, there is no stage 5.) He recorded one such encounter for each oncologist then cajoled them all into attending a communication skills lecture. Meanwhile, he selected snippets of conversation to splice into each physician's CD-ROM. The oncologists then reviewed the CD-ROM, and Tulsky recorded a second encounter.

What Tulsky found was truly impressive. After reviewing the CD-ROM, oncologists were now more than twice as likely to acknowledge and respond to patients' expressions of negative emotions as they had before. Armed with tips on how to respond to their patients' emotional pain, they no longer scurried away from each grimace or each plea for help. Given a chance to hear themselves struggling with their own patients, in the context of receiving advice about how to handle just such situations, these oncologists were now better prepared to recognize and respond in such situations in the future. Tulsky had proven that it's never too late to improve a physician's bedside manner.

Indeed, the oncologists in Tulsky's study were no strangers to patients with negative emotions. They weren't green medical students reflexively panicking at the first sign that their patients were panicking. These were experienced oncologists, men and women who had taken care of hundreds of dying patients. They had spent thousands of hours talking with suffering patients, yet until they spent a few hours with Tulsky's intervention, many of them were at a loss as to how to respond when their patients pleaded for help.

It was brilliant, really. Give doctors a chance to see themselves through the eyes of a communication specialist and they quickly improve their performance. Think how much more prepared those oncologists will now be to teach these skills to their trainees. As Yogi Berra is reported to have said, "You can observe a lot by watching."

Tulsky and his colleagues have demonstrated that it's never too late to retrain experienced clinicians. After all, most of us doctors want to improve ourselves. That's why we read medical journals throughout our careers. We don't become physicians by expecting the medical world to stand still. And most of us recognize that the softer side of our jobs—talking to patients from so many different backgrounds, each one with a different set of clinical problems—is incredibly challenging to master. Almost all of us will admit to struggling with how to handle unhappy patients. Consequently, many of us are receptive when people like Tulsky give us practical advice for how to improve our communication.

We have the will, and now people like Tulsky are showing us the way. To build on this new way, we need to put programs like Tulsky's on steroids—bulk them up and put them to work. We need to make specialty recertification contingent upon completing communication training.

But how do we convince the powers that be to make such training a standard part of medical education? Time, once again, to call in the lawyers.

MALPRACTICE FOR MISCOMMUNICATION

The MAG Mutual Insurance Company calls it MMS—medical mal-practice stress—the painful emotions physicians experience after they have been named in a malpractice suit. The physicians I have spoken with who have been named in lawsuits describe their experience in court as the worst time of their professional lives, even if they are ultimately exonerated. Just being sued is so traumatizing that if you search the Internet today, you will find a whole range of organizations and companies set up to help physicians cope with the emotional af-termath of malpractice litigation. It is safe to say that physicians are highly motivated to do what they can, whatever they can to avoid malpractice suits. Many simply work as hard as they can to provide good medical care, thereby hoping to avoid the mistakes that would compel someone to take them to court. Others respond to their fear of malpractice by ordering unnecessary tests and procedures on their patients, mistakenly believing that such aggressive care will reduce their chance of being sued. But there is a better way to avoid lawsuits, and one that may convince all of these former biology and chemistry majors to take the behavioral sciences more seriously.

Research on malpractice suits has shown that the law typically comes down hardest on physicians who lack empathy. That means that interventions like the one developed by Tulsky may end up be-coming a routine part of medical education not because physicians demand such training in order to be more in tune with their patients' needs, but because physicians want to avoid lawsuits.

Let's start with a simple fact about malpractice litigation in the United States (where such lawsuits run rampant compared to other developed countries). Malpractice lawsuits do not successfully target poor technical care. When a team of Harvard researchers pored over medical charts, looking for examples of medical errors that had caused patients harm, they found that malpractice lawsuits didn't successfully target these errors. One patient might develop a urinary infection while in the hospital, for example, because the physician left a urinary catheter in the patient's bladder too long. Another might experience such an infection despite no evidence of negligent care. The Harvard researchers discovered that lawsuits were just as likely to target technically good physicians as technically bad ones. A patient whose infection was directly attributable to bad medical care was no more likely to sue the hospital than one whose infection was a consequence of bad luck.

Then why do lawsuits happen? What causes one patient to sue their doctor and another to let things slide? You guessed it, communication! In a groundbreaking study, Wendy Levinson, a physician at the University of Toronto, tape-recorded two groups of physicians— one group, after many years of practice, had never been sued; another group had been sued two or more times. She and her team then analyzed the physicians' respective communication styles, whether the physicians responded to patient utterances with supportive comments like "uh-huh" and "I see," for example, and whether the doctors expressed signs of empathy and understanding. From these analyses, Levinson discovered a canyon-size divide—physicians who had been sued performed significantly worse on all of these communication measures.

In another analysis of the same recordings, Levinson took things a step further, placing a voice filter over the recording so that her coders could no longer hear the physicians' words clearly. Instead, the researchers confined their analysis to the tone of the physicians' voices, over a mere ten seconds of the encounter. Was the voice hard and monotone or gentle and expressive? Those physicians who'd been sued demonstrated much harsher and less sympathetic tones, their voices signifying dominance rather than partnership.

These doctors weren't being sued because they were making medical errors. They were being sued because they came across as jerks!

Empowered patients can't have true power, can't play an active role in important decisions, if they are met on the other end of the stethoscope by poor communicators. Those of us who care about shared decision making have been pushing for better communication lessons at medical schools and beyond. Perhaps now we will be joined by the large number of medical professionals interested in reducing malpractice claims.

DOOR HANDLE PROBLEM

"I do my best to educate my patients and help them make decisions. But good communication takes time. How do you expect busy clinicians to do all these things you're asking them to do?"

This is probably the most common line of questioning I encounter when talking with medical audiences. I appreciate how busy most doctors are, and I lament the crazy U.S. health-care system, which pays more money for family physicians to perform a five-minute skin biopsy than to spend twenty minutes discussing end-of-life concerns with their patients. But I disagree that good communication will necessarily eat up physicians' limited time. In many of the doctor–patient encounters I've listened to, I've noticed that physicians spend a tremendous amount of time talking to their patients in language that their patients don't understand. They'd probably be able to spend less time in such conversations if they communicated more effectively. In addition, when a patient they encounter is well informed, the discussion can proceed much more efficiently. One plastic surgeon I've spoken with created an online tool to help his patients understand their breast reconstruction alternatives. He soon discovered after implementing this tool that the average length of his clinic visits had declined.

When I lay out this reasoning for clinical audiences, I encounter mixed responses. Some heads bob up and down and others move side to side. That's when I pull out one more consideration, the door handle problem. This problem is familiar to every clinician, if not necessarily by that name. In a classic example of the phenomenon, I began one of my appointments by asking my patient, "How can I help you today?" The patient told me, "My knee hurts." I quickly began posing a series of yes-or-no inquiries ("Does your knee hurt at night? Does it hurt when you walk up stairs?"), followed by a focused clinical exam and a completion of the encounter. Glad that I had handled the patient's concerns in a timely manner, I reached for the door handle only to be interrupted by the concerned patient: "But what about my chest pain?" I sat back down in my chair and continued the appointment, knowing I would now fall even further behind in my clinic schedule.

Early in my career, I got angry about such door handle questions. I was irate that a patient had wasted my time on his knee problem when he had been harboring a life-threatening symptom like chest pain. Eventually (embarrassingly slowly), I realized that I should instead be angry with myself for such door handle surprises. The patient had had no way of knowing that his intermittent chest pain (which he had attributed to indigestion, not heart disease) was more serious than his constant knee pain (which was from good old-fashioned wear-and-tear arthritis). But I should have known not to drill down on a detailed history of his knee pain until after I had taken the time, early in the encounter, to elicit a fuller set of his concerns. My eagerness to move the encounter along had only succeeded in extending the visit.

The door handle problem resonates with physicians. They've all encountered door handle diagnoses and are eager to avoid more of them. They quickly recognize the value, in time as well as in medical care, of being a better communicator. The same goes for decision-making conversations. Good communication often takes less time than bad. When physicians don't elicit patients' questions and concerns early in a conversation, they head down dead-end paths, forced to retrace their conversational meanderings when patients finally get a chance to say what they care about. If physicians don't assess patient understanding in the course of a conversation, they risk wasting time explaining subsequent information. For the same reason most people can't learn calculus until they've learned algebra, most patients can't decide among their treatment alternatives until they understand their diagnoses.

ACHIEVING TRANSFORMATION

Susanne Petit was only twenty-seven weeks into her pregnancy when she went into labor, a terrifying situation for anyone but especially terrifying for Petit, who was only nineteen years old and whose labor was progressing so rapidly that she realized the baby would be delivered at home, far away from any kind of medical assistance. The ambulance arrived shortly after she had given birth to her baby boy, and the EMTs immediately placed young Gabriel on a ventilator. The hospital's NICU team worked night and day to help Gabriel, but even three days into his life, his situation was tenuous. He had bled into his brain. His chances of survival were still good, but the likelihood that he would escape major neurologic damage was vanishing.

Dr. Annie Janvier came to talk with Gabriel's young parents, to explain his situation and to work with them to decide what to do next. After explaining the likelihood that Gabriel would have cerebral palsy, she began describing all the modern equipment that could help him nevertheless thrive. But before she could elaborate, Gabriel's father interrupted. "Will we be able to love him?" he asked.

She reassured him that he would. Gabriel's mother then asked, "Will he be able to love us?" Janvier explained that Gabriel would certainly have the kind of love for them that any child would have for his parents. Then Gabriel's father chimed in with an even stranger question: "Will he be able to have sex?"

Janvier was shocked. Their baby lay in the NICU, every orifice seemingly attached to a piece of high-tech medical equipment, and this dad was asking whether his son would be able to have erections? She struggled to stay calm and explained that all his body parts should be able to work fine but that, of course, to have sex he would need a partner and . . .

"So he will be able to get it up and do it himself if he wants to?"

The conversation was getting stranger by the minute. And then the father shifted gears and asked another bizarre question, seemingly out of left field. "Will he be able to make pizza?" he asked.

At this point in the conversation most physicians would doubt the competence of these parents to cope with the difficult life facing this child and question their ability to participate in the challenging decisions coming around the corner, tough decisions about whether to keep him on the ventilator, agonizing choices about whether to aggressively treat opportunistic infections. The Petits also had to figure out whether they were capable of caring for Gabriel at home or whether they would need to send him to a nursing facility.

So far in this chapter, I have discussed steps that health-care leaders need to take to better prepare physicians to interact with patients who want to play a role in their health-care decisions, from how medical leaders select and train medical students to how they retrain practicing physicians so that they will be better communicators. None of these measures are magic bullets. All will need to be improved over time, as we learn more about how to better identify promising medical talent and how to more effectively train physicians in the science of decision making. But we should not delay implementing these steps in anticipation of these improvements. We need to start taking these steps right away. We shouldn't let perfection be the enemy of progress. If we wait for interventions to be perfect before we implement them—DVDs and CD-ROMs that transform doctors and patients into communication gurus—we'll lose out on the chance of helping today's patients make better decisions and of helping today's doctors become better decision-making partners.

We now know that shared decision making won't happen unless we take further action to help patients and their doctors work together as partners. The end of the revolution is within our grasp. The only question is whether we will reach out to grab hold of our opportunity.

In the NICU that day, Janvier was not ready to give up on partnering with the Petits in making the difficult medical decisions facing them. She wasn't inclined to rush out of the room and start making decisions on her own. She didn't feel compelled to throw a dose of jargon at these overwhelmed parents in hopes of intimidating them into following her medical recommendations. Instead, she continued to try to understand this young couple. That's when Gabriel's father elaborated on his reason for asking about pizza. "My family has a pizza place. My uncle opened it. We both work there. So does my cousin Samuel, who is a mongol [was born with Down syndrome]. Samuel puts pepperoni on pizza. His father makes the dough. I deliver the pizza. Susanne answers the phone and serves at the tables. If our son is happy like Samuel and can work with us, he will be okay. We will be okay."

Janvier realized that the Petits had more knowledge of a life with a disabled child than she had realized. Gabriel's mother then continued explaining their background. "Our family lives together. We have the same routine every day: get up, go to the pizza joint, work together, eat together, come home, watch a film and eat pizza. Well, sometimes we eat something else! Then we go to bed and . . . well, um . . . you probably know already that we have sex. We don't have much money, but we have enough. If Gabriel can have the same life we have, he will be okay. We will be okay."

Pizza and sex. Very strange questions until this doctor took the time to understand where this family was coming from.

Revolutions are often fought over dichotomies—the king versus the people, the bourgeoisie versus the proletariat, and of course the autonomous patient versus the paternalistic physician. When Karen Ann Quinlan lay in a hospital bed tethered to a ventilator against her parents' wishes, society was truly torn about who had the right to decide her fate. Some people believed that patients and their families had a duty to follow doctors' orders, convinced that decisions about ventilators were beyond the reach of laypeople. They contended that patients only needed whatever information doctors deemed necessary to convince them to follow the appropriate plan.

But the revolutionaries had different ideas. Power, they argued, belongs to patients; information is a necessity. The goal of medical care should be to pave the way for activated patients, ready now to make their own medical decisions. Or as my sixth grader would put it, autonomy rules, paternalism drools!

So the revolutionaries toppled the old guard. They threw out the idea of the all-knowing, ever-powerful physician. But they didn't have new leaders ready to step up in their place. They didn't have an army of new physicians in the wings, prepared to welcome newly activated patients. Physicians' lack of readiness may not have mattered, however, because few patients were prepared for the revolution. To this day many patients, especially those with symptomatic acute illnesses, don't want to be activated; they want to be cured. And while in the abstract they want to be informed about their illnesses, many don't know what to do with this information.

Response from many leaders of the patient-empowerment revolution has been to double down on autonomy. Bioethicist Art Caplan describes their doubling down in vivid terms: "The Freddy Krueger of bioethics for the better part of two decades has been the doctor who pushes his or her values onto the patient . . . This devil has been completely exorcised, and a large part of contemporary bioethics scholarship has been devoted to the task of assuring that the paternalistic doctor stays dead and buried." Not exactly the image of a revolution that has settled into a calm new order. Indeed, some revolutionaries contend that the only way to assure the continued death of the paternalistic physician is for patients to grab full hold of the decision-making power. As one leading scholar put it, the self-governing person "makes decisions for him- or herself." Thus, deferring to physicians is an abdication of the patient's duty: "In turning over a major health-care decision to another, a patient does not meet that ideal of self-determination." By this logic, autonomy is not just a patient's right; it is his or her duty.

This insistence on patient-dominated decision making has predictably been met with backlash, with opposing scholars arguing that the pendulum has swung too far in the direction of autonomy. Lawyer and bioethicist Carl Schneider contends that "many people do not hunger to make their own medical decisions." They even have "substantial reasons for forgoing medical decisions, reasons which make it more plausible that they truly wish to forgo them." Schneider's arguments, which I'm largely sympathetic to, have been met by a certain amount of scorn, the specter of Freddy Krueger rising from the dead being too much for some revolutionaries to swallow.

And so it goes, the back and forth between autonomy and paternalism: argue, argue; debate, debate; moral, immoral; ethical, unethical. How will the debate end? With understanding. The real borderline between moral and immoral is not the divide between autonomy and paternalism but rather the space between empathy and obliviousness.

Educating patients about clinical facts won't, alone, empower patients to integrate these facts with their values to make autonomous health-care decisions. Teaching them that they have a right to participate in their health care won't necessarily cause them to participate. Educating doctors about their duty to involve patients in medical decisions won't necessarily work either. We've been lecturing medical students about autonomy and ethics for a couple of decades now, and we've reached the limits of that approach.

It is time to move from power struggles to power sharing. If physicians and patients learn to communicate better with each other, they can figure out the best decisions together. If at the end of such conversations the patient chooses, it will likely be a choice that has been better informed by the doctor's perspective. If the conversation ends instead with a patient accepting a doctor's recommendation, that advice will more likely reflect the patient's preferences. At the end of the day, isn't that what the revolution has always strived for?

I opened this book with a story about Fred Furelli, a patient thrown into insomnia by a difficult decision about how to treat his newly diagnosed prostate cancer. Torn by indecision, he asked for my advice and I refused to give it. I told you how that story began, how I bungled the conversation with my awkward figure-skating analogy. But I didn't tell you how it ended.

Not surprisingly, Furelli didn't respond to my figure-skating comment by becoming an empowered patient. He dismissed my analogy and asked again for my advice. But I didn't accede to his request; I spoke with him for a while longer, to get a better sense of his preferences. Only when I felt that I understood him did I make a recommendation: "I think you should have surgery."

He paused for a moment. "Oh gosh, the thought of them cutting into my body . . ."

We talked a bit longer. Then, when I thought I understood him better, I offered up radiation as a nonsurgical alternative. He fretted over the side effects. We talked about those for a while, and it was clear that he understood that surgery would cause many of the same side effects. At some point I recommended watchful waiting too, and he bemoaned the passivity of this approach.

My recommendations clearly didn't come off sounding like dogmatic, doctorly determinations given how readily Furelli rejected them. The whole interaction felt more like a changing room in a department store, a chance for him to try on different choices to see what felt best. Eventually, I returned to one of my earlier recommendations and it finally felt to him like a good fit. "You're right, Doc. That's the best choice for me. Thanks for your help. I couldn't have done it without you."

I'd taken the time to try to understand his preferences and had taken the weight off his shoulders by framing the conversation in a series of soft recommendations. His responses to my recommendations gave me a chance to help him understand his own preferences more clearly. Ultimately, I'm not sure which one of us made the decision that day. But I think we made the right choice.

Acknowledgments

I tell a lot of stories in *Critical Decisions,* many about my own clinical practice and some about my life and the lives of people close to me. I must start right off, then, thanking all of the people I have learned from along the way whose stories I have shared. Although I have changed the names of the patients I write about in *Critical Decisions,* if they recognize themselves in these pages I hope they know I am grateful to them all. It really is an honor to practice medicine and help people through what are often the most difficult parts of their lives.

I tell some other people's stories here too. Some of those stories were published in articles and books, and I have listed those publications in the selected bibliography. But other people shared their stories with me in interviews and less formal conversations, and I thank all of those people for giving me their perspectives.

I write about a lot of "my own" research in this book, and here I have to acknowledge that most of the "I"s I use in discussing my experiments and other studies are really "we"s. I have been lucky to collaborate with many wonderful people in my career. I was mentored by some amazing people early on, people like Mark Siegler, Bob Arnold, George Loewenstein, and David Asch, all of whom helped me begin to sort out the complex world of ethics and decision making. I've also learned a lot from those people I have mentored, especially Angie Fagerlin and Brian Zikmund-Fisher, who have easily taught me as much as I've taught them. I've had too many collaborators to mention them all by name here in the acknowledgments, but you know who you are and now I hope you realize how indebted I am to all of you for turning my crazy ideas into legitimate science.

Thanks, too, to the people and organizations that have been generous enough to fund my edgy research over the years. (I prefer "edgy" to "weird," just like I prefer being called "sinewy" to "skinny," but I will let you decide which, if any, of these words apply to either my research or me.) I have received lots of research support from the Department of Veterans Affairs over the years, and of course I have also had the pleasure of practicing medicine in that amazing healthcare system. I have received over a decade and a half of support from the National Institutes of Health to study topics like shared decision making; thanks to Wendy Nelson at the National Cancer Institute for all of her help over the years. And I have also received support these last few years from the Robert Wood Johnson Foundation through its wonderful Investigator Awards in Health Policy Research. All healthcare policies eventually end up working, or failing, at the bedside. So if we want better policies, we need to understand how doctors and patients make medical decisions together.

Thanks to those of you who read drafts of this book: Lawrence Ngo, James Tulsky, Jack Fowler, Jeff Belkora, and Rita Ouseph. Special thanks to Andrea Angott, Kath Pollak, Angie Fagerlin, and Clara Lee for slogging through multiple chapters in draft form. Thanks to Karan Chhabra and Janet Schwartz for sharing examples of doctor–patient encounters that they have listened to in the course of their research. Much gratitude to Katija Waldrop, Chulpan Khismatova, Emily Cao, Evan Tsun, Lillie Williamson, and Katlego Modiselle for helping me put together the manuscript.

Jim Levine, of the Levine Greenberg Literary Agency, is a wonderful agent who helped me take a bare-bones idea and turn it into a presentable proposal. And then he did an even bigger favor and helped me find a wonderful editor at HarperOne, Jeanette Perez, who has been a complete joy to work with.

And finally to my wife, Paula. Thanks for being an even bigger part of this book than either of us had planned. You are way cool, girl. This book is dedicated to you.

Eight Tips to Help You and Your Doctor Make Better Decisions Together

Shared decision making depends on good communication from both ends of the stethoscope. People like me are working to make doctors better prepared to work with prepared patients. You can help us do this by seeking out doctors who are good communicators and by lobbying your local hospital or medical clinic to start offering decision aids to patients. Meanwhile, here are eight things you can do to increase the chance that when you face critical medical decisions, you will be able to partner with your health-care providers to make better choices.

1. Recognize that you, the patient, have a role to play in your decisions.

The "right" medical choice frequently depends on your preferences—on what *you* care about. Many health-care choices involve trade-offs, with one set of pros and cons pitted against another. Consequently, the best choice will often differ from one patient to another, depending on what each patient thinks and feels about these trade-offs. Making medical decisions starts with the realization that the right choice is not simply a question of the medical facts but depends upon your values.

2. Realize that you are not alone.

Being an "empowered patient" doesn't mean being alone in making a final decision. It is okay to ask for your doctor's advice. Don't be hesitant to lean on friends and family for guidance. You are not alone. The best choices often depend on teamwork.

3. Get informed about your alternatives.

Whether you want to be the decision maker of last resort or prefer to follow your doctor's advice, you will usually be happier about your decision if you learn about your alternatives. Find out if there is a decision aid relevant to your choice. The University of Ottawa (www .decisionaid.ohri.ca) and the Informed Medical Decisions Foundation (www.informedmedicaldecisions.org) have excellent websites providing information about available decision aids for various diagnoses. Find out if your hospital or medical clinic has a decision-coaching service. If it doesn't, politely ask why not (they won't change their ways without an occasional nudge), and see if they will find a nursing student, medical student, or other health-care trainee to accompany you to your doctor appointments.

4. Be an active listener.

Is your doctor talking too fast? Speaking in words you can't comprehend? Be prepared to ask for clarification. Whenever possible, come to your appointment with a list of questions. If you are shy, bring someone to your appointment who can take notes and who's not afraid to ask questions. Don't be afraid to tell your doctor when you are confused. And remember, if you don't express your bewilderment, your doctor is probably going to assume that everything is okay. It is not rude to ask the doctor to take time to explain things again. That is what doctors are paid to do.

5. Communicate what you care about.

Even if you plan on letting your doctor make critical decisions for you, you should do what you can to help your doctor give you good advice. If your doctor doesn't understand what you care about, then it will be difficult for her to recommend a choice that best fits your preferences. Would you rather have surgery in order to make a permanent health change, or are you deathly afraid of surgery and would rather take daily medications to control a problem? Either way, your doctor should know what you prefer.

6. If you have time to decide, then take your time.

Sometimes the best way to avoid bad decisions is to take a tincture of time, time in which you can sleep on your decision (research has shown that even when we are not aware of it, our brains continue to unconsciously ponder our decisions) and also time during which strong emotions have a chance to subside. If you do not know how much time you have to make a decision, try to find out. A hint: If you are not in the hospital, you probably have time for a second opinion. And you almost certainly have time to search the Internet or ask your computer-savvy cousin to search the Internet for you.

7. Seek out help from other patients.

When you are forced to imagine the unimaginable ("What will my life be like if they amputate my leg?"), seek out people who are in that situation and ask them about their lives. And remember, when they tell you that they are happier than you imagine you could be in that situation, it is probably your imagination that is letting you down. People are usually better at emotionally adapting to difficult circumstances than they imagine they will be.

8. Stay informed.

Keep visiting the Critical Decisions part of my website (www .peterubel.com). I will keep on unearthing decision-making lessons and posting them there, with responses from all of you. That way none of us have to figure these things out on our own.

Selected Bibliography

"I really enjoyed your book," my law professor friend told me after reading one of my previous tomes, "but I wish you had listed more of your references." Such is the academic way: Every statement, no matter how apparent, needs to be supported by a reference.[1] I will no doubt disappoint this law professor once again with my *Critical Decisions* bibliography, because I have chosen to only list major works crucial to understanding the points I make in each chapter. If I discuss a study or an experiment, I will cite it here in the list of references. But I do not pretend to cite every work that has influenced my thinking on all of the topics I cover in this book. For starters, I don't want to try your patience. More importantly, I have a terrible memory for that kind of stuff.

A quick word on all of the quotations I use in the book, in telling stories about doctors and patients. When these conversations came from my own experience, these quotes are not verbatim. I didn't tape-record my own visits and so I am relying on my imperfect memory to portray the gist of the story. By contrast, when the quotes came from tape-recorded conversations of doctor–patient encounters, I not only made sure to mention that these are from tape-recorded encounters, but I also made sure that the words in the quotes are verbatim—just how it happened, baby!

Prologue

Annas, G. J. *The Rights of Patients: The Basic ACLU Guide to Patient Rights.* Totowa, NJ: Humana Press, 1992.
Beauchamp, T. L., and J. F. Childress. *Principles of Biomedical Ethics.* New York: Oxford Univ. Press, 1994.

---

1. I should, for instance, have referenced this statement!

Fischhoff, B. "Value Elicitation: Is There Anything in There?" *American Psychologist* 46, no. 8 (1991): 835–847.

Groopman, Jerome. Interview by Stephen Colbert. *The Colbert Report.* Comedy Central, October 3, 2011. http://www.colbertnation.com/the-colbert-report-videos/398786/october–03–2011/jerome-groopman

Katz, J. *The Silent World of Doctor and Patient.* New York: Free Press, 1984.

McNeil, B. J., et al. "On the Elicitation of Preferences for Alternative Therapies." *New England Journal of Medicine* 306, no. 21 (1982): 1259–1262.

Miles, J. "Protecting Patient Self-Determination: New Legislation Requires Healthcare Providers to Inform Patients of Rights Regarding Advance Directives." *Health Progress* 72, no. 3 (1991): 26–30.

Schneider, C. E. *The Practice of Autonomy: Patients, Doctors, and Medical Decisions.* New York: Oxford Univ. Press, 1998.

Tversky, A., and E. Shafir. "Choice Under Conflict: The Dynamics of Deferred Choice." *Psychological Science* 3, no. 6 (1992): 358–361.

Chapter 1: When Doctor Knew Best

I can think of no better books to introduce readers to the history of "doctor knows best" than those listed below by Katz and Rothman. These academic books are quite readable for lay audiences and are bursting with telling details. Lerner's book on breast cancer treatment is another fine example of academic writing that deserves a broad audience.

Fitts, William T., Jr. and I. S. Ravdin. "What Philadelphia Physicians Tell Patients with Cancer." *Journal of the American Medical Association* 153, no. 10 (1953): 901–904.

"The First Family: Betty Ford: Facing Cancer." *TIME* 104, no. 15 (October 7, 1974).

Ford, B. *The Times of My Life.* New York: HarperCollins, 1978.

Jonas, H. "Philosophical Reflections on Experimenting with Human Subjects." *Daedalus* 98 (1969): 219–247.

Katz, J. *The Silent World of Doctor and Patient.* New York: Free Press, 1984.

Krugman, S. "Infectious Hepatitis: Detection of Virus During the Incubation Period and in Clinically Inapparent Infection." *New England Journal of Medicine* 261, no. 15 (1959): 729–734.

Leopold, E. *Under the Radar.* New Brunswick, NJ: Rutgers Univ. Press, 2008.

Lerner, B. H. *The Breast Cancer Wars: Hope, Fear, and the Pursuit of a Cure in Twentieth-Century America.* New York: Oxford Univ. Press, 2001.

Morris, A. J., et al. "Prevention of Rheumatic Fever by Treatment of Previous Streptococcic Infections." *Journal of the American Medical Association* 160, no. 2 (1956): 114–116.

Mukherjee, S. *The Emperor of All Maladies: A Biography of Cancer.* New York: Scribner, 2010.

Oken, D. "What to Tell Cancer Patients." *Journal of the American Medical Association* 175, no. 13 (1961): 1120–1961.

Porter, R. *The Greatest Benefit to Mankind: A Medical History of Humanity.* New York: W. W. Norton, 1999.

Rothman, D. J. *Strangers at the Bedside.* New York: Basic Books, 1991.

Shore, D. "Developing the 'Concept'." *House, M.D.* Fox Broadcasting, February 16, 2006. http://www.hulu.com/watch/21606/house-developing-the-concept.

Chapter 2: A Sleeping Girl Wakes Up a Profession

Much of the detail from this chapter came from Joseph and Julia Quinlan's touching telling of their story.

Andrews, K. "Persistent Vegetative State." *British Medical Journal* 303, no. 6794 (1991): 121.

Canterbury v. Spence, 464 F. 2d 772 (DC Cir. 1972).

"A Definition of Irreversible Coma." *Journal of the American Medical Association* 205, no. 6 (1968): 337–340.

Excerpts from Judge Muir's Decision in the Karen Ann Quinlan Case. *New York Times,* November 11, 1975.

Katz, J. *The Silent World of Doctor and Patient.* New York: Free Press, 1984.

"The Law: A Life in the Balance." *TIME* 106, no. 18 (November 3, 1975).

"The Law: The Right to Live—Or Die." *TIME* 106, no. 17 (October 27, 1975).

Lerner, B. H. *The Breast Cancer Wars: Hope, Fear, and the Pursuit of a Cure in Twentieth-Century America.* New York: Oxford Univ. Press, 2001.

Natanson v. Kline and St. Francis Hospital and School of Nursing, Inc. 186 Kan. 393, 350 P. 2nd 1093 (1960).

Quinlan, J., J. Quinlan, and P. Battelle. *Karen Ann: The Quinlans Tell Their Story.* New York: Doubleday, 1977.

Chapter 3: Lost in Translation

Arras, J. D. "Beyond Cruzan: Individual Rights, Family Autonomy, and the Persistent Vegetative State." *Journal of the American Geriatrics Society* 39, no. 10 (1991): 1018–1024.

Boyle, C. M. "Difference Between Patients' and Doctors' Interpretation of Some Common Medical Terms." *British Medical Journal* 2, no. 5704 (1970): 286–289.

Cassell, E. J. *Talking with Patients: Clinical Technique.* Cambridge, MA: MIT Press, 1985.

Castro, C. M., et al. "Babel Babble: Physicians' Use of Unclarified Medical Jargon with Patients." *American Journal of Health Behavior* 31, suppl. 1 (2007): S85–95.

Chapple, A., et al. "Clinical Terminology: Anxiety and Confusion Amongst Families Undergoing Genetic Counseling." *Patient Education and Counseling* 32, nos. 1–2 (1997): 81–91.

David, L. "The Pilot (Part 2)." *Seinfeld.* NBC, May 20, 1993.

Engel, K., et al. "Patient Comprehension of Emergency Department Care and Instructions: Are Patients Aware of When They Do Not Understand?" *Annals of Emergency Medicine* 53, no. 4 (2009): 454–461, e415.

Gilovich, T., et al. "The Spotlight Effect in Social Judgment: An Egocentric Bias in Estimates of the Salience of One's Own Actions and Appearance." *Journal of Personality and Social Psychology* 78, no. 2 (2000): 211–222.

Hadlow, J., and M. Pitts. "The Understanding of Common Health Terms by Doctors, Nurses, and Patients." *Social Science and Medicine* 32, no. 2 (1991): 193–196.

Korsch, B. M., et al. "Gaps in Doctor–Patient Communication." *Pediatrics* 42, no. 5 (1968): 855–871.

Lidz, C. W., et al. *Informed Consent: A Study of Decisionmaking in Psychiatry.* New York: Guilford Press, 1984.

Novack, D. H., et al. "Changes in Physicians' Attitudes Toward Telling the Cancer Patient." *Journal of the American Medical Association* 241, no. 9 (1979): 897–900.

Ogden, J., et al. "What's in a Name? An Experimental Study of Patients' Views of the Impact and Function of a Diagnosis." *Family Practice* 20, no. 3 (2003): 248–253.

Ross, L., et al. "The 'False Consensus Effect': An Egocentric Bias in Social Perception and Attribution Processes." *Journal of Experimental Social Psychology* 13, no. 3 (1977): 279–301.

Samora, J., et al. "Medical Vocabulary Knowledge Among Hospital Patients." *Journal of Health and Human Behavior* 2, no. 2 (1961): 83–92.

Schneider, C. E. *The Practice of Autonomy: Patients, Doctors, and Medical Decisions.* New York: Oxford Univ. Press, 1998.

Silver-Isenstadt, A., and P. A. Ubel. "Medical Student Name Tags: Identification or Obfuscation?" *Journal of General Internal Medicine* 12, no. 11 (1997): 669–671.

Veatch, R. M. *The Patient–Physician Relation: The Patient as Partner.* Bloomington: Indiana Univ. Press, 1991.

Chapter 4: Blind to Each Other's Emotions

Ainsworth-Vaughn, N. *Claiming Power in Doctor–Patient Talk.* New York: Oxford Univ. Press, 1998.

Anderson, W. G., et al. " 'What Concerns Me Is . . .' Expression of Emotion by Advanced Cancer Patients During Outpatient Visits." *Supportive Care in Cancer* 16, no. 7 (2008): 803–811.

Folkman, S., and J. T. Moskowitz. "Stress, Positive Emotion, and Coping." *Current Directions in Psychological Science* 9, no. 4 (2000): 115–118.

Freud, S. "Humour." In *Penguin Freud Library, Volume 14: Art and Literature.* Edited by Albert Dickson. Harmondsworth, Middlesex: Penguin Books, 1990.

Kennifer, S., et al. "Negative Emotions in Cancer Care: Do Oncologists' Responses Depend on Severity and Type of Emotion?" *Patient Education and Counseling* 76, no. 1 (2009): 51–56.

Lerner, B. H. *The Breast Cancer Wars: Hope, Fear, and the Pursuit of a Cure in Twentieth-Century America.* New York: Oxford Univ. Press, 2001.

Parsons, G. N., et al. "Between Two Worlds: Medical Student Perceptions of Humor and Slang in the Hospital Setting." *Journal of General Internal Medicine* 16, no. 8 (2001): 544–549.

Pollak, K. I., et al. "Oncologist Communication About Emotion During Visits with Patients with Advanced Cancer." *Journal of Clinical Oncology* 25, no. 36 (2007): 5748–5752.

Schneider, C. E. *The Practice of Autonomy: Patients, Doctors, and Medical Decisions.* New York: Oxford Univ. Press, 1998.

Silver-Isenstadt, A., and P. A. Ubel. "Medical Student Name Tags: Identification or Obfuscation?" *Journal of General Internal Medicine* 12, no. 11 (1997): 669–671.

Smith, A. C., III and S. Kleinman. "Managing Emotions in Medical School: Students' Contacts with the Living and the Dead." *Social Psychology Quarterly* 52, no. 1 (1989): 56–69.

Ubel, P. A. *You're Stronger than You Think: Tapping into the Secrets of Emotionally Resilient People.* New York: McGraw-Hill, 2006.

Ubel, P. A., et al. "Don't Ask, Don't Tell: A Change in Medical Student Attitudes After Obstetrics/Gynecology Clerkships Toward Seeking Consent for Pelvic Examinations on an Anesthetized Patient." *American Journal of Obstetrics and Gynecology* 188, no. 2 (2003): 575–579.

Yoels, W. C., and J. M. Clair. "Laughter in the Clinic: Humor as Social Organization." *Symbolic Interaction* 18, no. 1 (1995): 39–58.

Chapter 5: Misimagining the Unimaginable

For a fuller account of how, why, and even whether people emotionally adapt to chronic illness and disability, you can read one of my earlier books. *You're Stronger than You Think* is a book I hope gains new popularity in the wake of the (no doubt) huge success of *Critical Decisions*.

Brickman, P., et al. "Lottery Winners and Accident Victims: Is Happiness Relative?" *Journal of Personality and Social Psychology* 36, no. 8 (1978): 917–927.

Carstensen, L. L. "Evidence for a Life-Span Theory of Socioemotional Selectivity." *Current Directions in Psychological Science* 4, no. 5 (1995): 151–156.

Fleming, C., et al. "A Decision Analysis of Alternative Treatment Strategies for Clinically Localized Prostate Cancer. Prostate Patient Outcomes Research Team." *Journal of the American Medical Association* 269, no. 20 (1993): 2650–2658.

Gilbert, D. T., et al. "Immune Neglect: A Source of Durability Bias in Affective Forecasting." *Journal of Personality and Social Psychology* 75, no. 3 (1998): 617–638.

Lacey, H. P., et al. "Hope I Die Before I Get Old: Mispredicting Happiness Across the Lifespan." *Journal of Happiness Studies* 7, no. 2 (2006): 167–182.

Loewenstein, G., and D. Schkade. "Wouldn't It Be Nice? Predicting Future Feelings." In *Well-Being: The Foundations of Hedonic Psychology.* Edited by D. Kahneman, E. Diener, and N. Schwarz. New York: Russell Sage Foundation, 1999.

Raiffa, H. *Decision Analysis.* Reading, MA: Addison-Wesley, 1968.

Riis, J., et al. "Ignorance of Hedonic Adaptation to Hemo-Dialysis: A Study Using Ecological Momentary Assessment." *Journal of Experimental Psychology: General* 134, no. 1 (2005): 3–9.

Ross, M. "Relation of Implicit Theories to the Construction of Personal Histories." *Psychological Review* 96, no. 2 (1989): 341–357.

Schkade, D. A., and D. Kahneman. "Does Living in California Make People Happy? A Focusing Illusion in Judgments of Life Satisfaction." *Psychological Science* 9, no. 5 (1998): 340–346.

Smith, D. M., et al. "Misremembering Colostomies? Former Patients Give Lower Utility Ratings than Do Current Patients." *Health Psychology* 25, no. 6 (2006): 688–695.

Ubel, P. *Free Market Madness: Why Human Nature Is at Odds with Economics—and Why It Matters.* Boston: Harvard Business Press, 2009.

Ubel, P. A., et al. "Whose Quality of Life? A Commentary Exploring Discrepancies Between Health State Evaluations of Patients and the General Public." *Quality of Life Research* 12, no. 6 (2003): 599–607.

Ubel, P. A., et al. "Misimagining the Unimaginable: The Disability Paradox and Healthcare Decision Making." *Health Psychology* 24, no. 4 suppl. (2005): S57-S62.

Wilkerson, M. *Amazing Journey: The Life of Pete Townshend.* Raleigh, NC: Lulu Press, 2006.

———. *Who Are You: The Life of Pete Townshend.* New York: Omnibus Press, 2008.

Wilson, K. A., et al. "Perception of Quality of Life by Patients, Partners, and Treating Physicians." *Quality of Life Research* 9, no. 9 (2000): 1041–1052.

Wilson, T. D., et al. "Focalism: A Source of Durability Bias in Affective Forecasting." *Journal of Personality and Social Psychology* 78, no. 5 (2000): 821–836.

Chapter 6: Beyond the Numbers

Karan Chhabra let me read his absolutely amazing undergraduate honors thesis from his senior year at Duke, and I quote from one of those conversations in this chapter.

Amsterlaw, J., et al. "Can Avoidance of Complications Lead to Biased Healthcare Decisions?" *Judgment and Decision Making* 1, no. 1 (2006): 64–75.

Angott, A., and P. Ubel. Unpublished research, 2011.

Chandler, J., and N. Schwarz. "How Extending Your Middle Finger Affects Your Perception of Others: Learned Movements Influence Concept Accessibility." *Journal of Experimental Social Psychology* 45, no. 1 (2009): 123–128.

Damasio, A. R. *Descartes' Error: Emotion, Reason, and the Human Brain.* New York: G. P. Putnam's Sons, 1994.

Fagerlin, A., et al. "Women's Decisions Regarding Tamoxifen for Breast Cancer Prevention: Responses to a Tailored Decision Aid." *Breast Cancer Research and Treatment* 119, no. 3 (2010): 613–620.

Fagerlin, A., et al. "How Making a Risk Estimate Can Change the Feel of That Risk: Shifting Attitudes Toward Breast Cancer Risk in a General Public Survey." *Patient Education and Counseling* 57, no. 3 (2005): 294–299.

Fagerlin, A., et al. " 'If I'm Better than Average, Then I'm OK?': Comparative Information Influences Beliefs About Risk and Benefits." *Patient Education and Counseling* 69, nos. 1–3 (2007): 140–144.

Fisher, B., et al. "Tamoxifen for the Prevention of Breast Cancer: Current Status of the National Surgical Adjuvant Breast and Bowel Project P–1 Study." *Journal of the National Cancer Institute* 97, no. 22 (2005): 1652–1662.

Hsee, C. K., et al. "Preference Reversals Between Joint and Separate Evaluations of Options: A Review and Theoretical Analysis." *Psychological Bulletin* 125, no. 5 (1999): 576–590.

Lerman, C., et al. "Controlled Trial of Pretest Education Approaches to Enhance Informed Decision-Making for BRCA1 Gene Testing." *Journal of the National Cancer Institute* 89, no. 2 (1997): 148–157.

Loewenstein, G. F., et al. "Risk as Feelings." *Psychological Bulletin* 127, no. 2 (2001): 267–286.

Peters, E., et al. "Numeracy and Decision Making." *Psychological Science* 17, no. 5 (2006): 407–413.

Rottenstreich, Y., and C. K. Hsee. "Money, Kisses, and Electric Shocks: On the Affective Psychology of Risk." *Psychological Science* 12, no. 3 (2001): 185–190.

Schwartz, L. M., et al. "The Role of Numeracy in Understanding the Benefit of Screening Mammography." *Annals of Internal Medicine* 127, no. 11 (1997): 966–972.

Schwarz, N. "When Thinking Feels Difficult: Meta-Cognitive Experiences in Judgment and Decision Making." *Medical Decision Making* 25, no. 1 (2005): 105–112.

Schwarz, N., and F. Strack. "Reports of Subjective Well-Being: Judgmental Processes and Their Methodological Implications." In *Well-Being: The Foundations of Hedonic Psychology.* Edited by D. Kahneman, E. Diener, and N. Schwarz. New York: Russell Sage Foundation, 1999.

Slovic, P., M. L. Finucane, E. Peters, and D. G. MacGregor. "Risk as Analysis and Risk as Feelings: Some Thoughts About Affect, Reason, Risk, and Rationality." *Risk Analysis* 24, no. 2 (2004): 311–322.

Song, H., and N. Schwarz. "If It's Difficult to Pronounce, It Must Be Risky." *Psychological Science* 20, no. 2 (2009): 135–138.

Ubel, P. A. "Is Information Always a Good Thing? Helping Patients Make 'Good' Decisions." *Medical Care* 40, no. 9, suppl. (2002): 39–44.

Ubel, P. A., et al. "Physicians Recommend Different Treatments for Patients than They Would Choose for Themselves." *Archives of Internal Medicine* 171, no. 7 (2011): 630–634.

Zikmund-Fisher, B. J., et al. "'Is 28% Good or Bad?': Evaluability and Preference Reversals in Health Care Decisions." *Medical Decision Making* 24, no. 2 (2004): 142–148.

Zikmund-Fisher, B. J., et al. "Risky Feelings: Why a 6% Risk of Cancer Does Not Always Feel Like 6%." *Patient Education and Counseling* 81, suppl. 1 (2010): S87-S93.

Chapter 7: Back and Forth over Life and Death

Nicholas Christakis is a physician and sociologist at Harvard who has received a lot of attention in recent years for his pioneering research on the social contagion of everything from obesity to happiness. But his early research on the art of prognostication in medical practice is equally impressive, and his book *Death Foretold* should be (here comes the cliché) required reading in medical and nursing schools.

Code of Medical Ethics of the American Medical Association. Chicago: American Medical Association Press, 1847.

Cassell, E. J. *Talking with Patients: Clinical Technique.* Cambridge, MA: MIT Press, 1985.

Christakis, N. A. *Death Foretold: Prophecy and Prognosis in Medical Care.* Chicago: Univ. of Chicago Press, 1999.

David, L. "The Pilot (Part 1)." *Seinfeld.* NBC, May 20, 1993.

Fagerlin, A., et al. "Cure Me Even If It Kills Me: Preferences for Invasive Cancer Treatment." *Medical Decision Making* 25, no. 6 (2005): 614–619.

Fins, J. J. "The Patient Self-Determination Act and Patient–Physician Collaboration in New York State." *New York State Journal of Medicine* 92, no. 11 (1992): 489–493.

Freeborne, N., J. Lynn, and N. A. Desbiens. "SUPPORT: Study to Understand Prognoses and Preferences for Outcomes and Risks of Treatments. Study Design." *Journal of Clinical Epidemiology* 43, suppl. (1990): 1S–123S.

Gould, S. J., et al. *The Richness of Life: The Essential Stephen Jay Gould.* New York: W. W. Norton, 2006.

Lamont, E. B., and N. A. Christakis. "Prognostic Disclosure to Patients with Cancer near the End of Life." *Annals of Internal Medicine* 134, no. 12 (1996): 1096–1105.

Percival, T. *Medical Ethics; Or, a Code of Institutes and Precepts, Adapted to the Professional Conduct of Physicians and Surgeons.* London: S. Russell for J. Johnson, 1803.

Spranca, M., et al. "Omission and Commission in Judgment and Choice." *Journal of Experimental Social Psychology* 27, no. 1 (1991): 76–105.

Weinstein, N. D. "Unrealistic Optimism About Susceptibility to Health Problems." *Journal of Behavioral Medicine* 5, no. 4 (1982): 441–460.

Chapter 8: Getting Good Advice

Baylis, F., and J. Downie. "Professional Recommendations: Disclosing Facts and Values." *Journal of Medical Ethics* 27, no. 1 (2001): 20–24.

Beisswanger, A. H., et al. "Risk Taking in Relationships: Differences in Deciding for Oneself Versus for a Friend." *Basic and Applied Social Psychology* 25, no. 2 (2003): 121–135.

Blackhall, L. J. "Must We Always Use CPR?" *New England Journal of Medicine* 317, no. 20 (1987): 1281–1285.

Fisher, S. "Institutional Authority and the Structure of Discourse." *Discourse Processes* 7, no. 2 (1984): 201–224.

Fowler, F. J., Jr., et al. "Comparison of Recommendations by Urologists and Radiation Oncologists for Treatment of Clinically Localized Prostate Cancer." *Journal of the American Medical Association* 283, no. 24 (2000): 3217–3222.

Gilovich, T., and V. H. Medvec. "The Experience of Regret: What, When, and Why." *Psychological Review* 102, no. 2 (1995): 379–395.

Gurmankin, A. D., et al. "The Role of Physicians' Recommendations in Medical Treatment Decisions." *Medical Decision Making* 22, no. 3 (2002): 262–271.

Kray, L., and R. Gonzalez. "Differential Weighting in Choice Versus Advice: I'll Do This, You Do That." *Journal of Behavioral Decision Making* 12, no. 3 (1999): 207–217.

Meier, B. "Sales Tactics on Implants Raise Doubts." *New York Times,* June 1, 2011. New York edition p. B1.

Quill, T. E., and H. Bordy. "Physician Recommendations and Patient Autonomy: Finding a Balance Between Physician Power and Patient Choice." *Annals of Internal Medicine* 125, no. 9 (1996): 763–769.

Quinlan, J., J. Quinlan, and P. Battelle. *Karen Ann: The Quinlans Tell Their Story.* New York: Doubleday, 1977.

Siminoff, L. A., and J. H. Fetting. "Effects of Outcome Framing on Treatment Decisions in the Real World: Impact of Framing on Adjuvant Breast Cancer Decisions." *Medical Decision Making* 9, no. 4 (1989): 262–271.

Ubel, P. A. "'What Should I Do, Doc?': Some Psychologic Benefits of Physician Recommendations." *Archives of Internal Medicine* 162, no. 9 (2002): 977–980.

Ubel, P. A., et al. "Physicians Recommend Different Treatments for Patients than They Would Choose for Themselves." *Archives of Internal Medicine* 171, no. 7 (2011): 630–634.

Veatch, R. "Ethical Medicine in a Revolutionary Age." *Hastings Center Report* 2, no. 3 (1972): 3–6.

Chapter 9: Empowering Patients with Information

Jack Fowler was generous enough to let me interview him so he could tell me stories about the birth of the decision-aid movement.

Barry, M. J., et al. "A Randomized Trial of a Multimedia Shared Decision-Making Program for Men Facing a Treatment Decision for Benign Prostatic Hyperplasia." *Disease Management and Clinical Outcomes* 1, no. 1 (1997): 5–14.

Brownlee, S. *Overtreated: Why Too Much Medicine Is Making Us Sicker and Poorer.* New York: Bloomsbury, 2008.

McPherson, K., et al. "Small-Area Variations in the Use of Common Surgical Procedures: An International Comparison of New England, England, and Norway." *New England Journal of Medicine* 307, no. 21 (1982): 1310–1314.

O'Connor, A., et al. "Do Patient Decision Aids Meet Effectiveness Criteria of the International Patient Decision Aid Standards Collaboration? A Systematic Review and Meta-Analysis." *Medical Decision Making* 27, no. 5 (2007): 554–574.

Peele, P., et al. "Decreased Use of Adjuvant Breast Cancer Therapy in a Randomized Controlled Trial of a Decision Aid with Individualized Risk Information." *Medical Decision Making* 25, no. 3 (2005): 301–307.

Wennberg, J., and A. Gittelsohn. "Small Area Variations in Health Care Delivery." *Science* 182, no. 4117 (1973): 1102–1108.

Wennberg, J. E. "Improving the Medical Decision-Making Process." *Health Affairs* 7, no. 1 (1988): 99–106.

———. *Tracking Medicine: A Researcher's Quest to Understand Health Care.* New York: Oxford Univ. Press, 2010.

Wennberg, J. E., and F. J. Fowler. "A Test of Consumer Contribution to Small Area Variations in Health Care Delivery." *Journal of the Maine Medical Association* 68, no. 8 (1977): 275–279.

Chapter 10: Aligning Information with Behavior

Denes-Raj, V., et al. "The Generality of the Ratio–Bias Phenomenon." *Personality and Social Psychology Bulletin* 21, no. 10 (1995): 1083–1092.

Fagerlin, A., et al. "Reducing the Influence of Anecdotal Reasoning on People's Health Care Decisions: Is a Picture Worth a Thousand Statistics?" *Medical Decision Making* 25, no. 4 (2005): 398–405.

Hawley, S. T., et al. "The Impact of the Format of Graphical Presentation on Health-Related Knowledge and Treatment Choices." *Patient Education and Counseling* 73, no. 3 (2008): 448–455.

Nisbett, R., and L. Ross. *Human Inference: Strategies and Shortcomings of Social Judgment.* Englewood Cliffs, NJ: Prentice-Hall, 1980.

Peters, E., et al. "Numeracy and Decision Making." *Psychological Science* 17, no. 5 (2006): 407–413.

Ubel, P. A., et al. "Testing Whether Decision Aids Introduce Cognitive Biases: Results of a Randomized Trial." *Patient Education and Counseling* 80, no. 2 (2010): 158–163.

Ubel, P. A., et al. "The Inclusion of Patient Testimonials in Decision Aids: Effects on Treatment Choices." *Medical Decision Making* 21, no. 1 (2001): 60–68.

Volandes, A. E., et al. "Video Decision Support Tool for Advance Care Planning in Dementia: Randomised Controlled Trial." *British Medical Journal* 338, no. b2159 (2009).

Zikmund-Fisher, B., et al. "Alternate Methods of Framing Information About Medication Side Effects: Incremental Risk Versus Total Risk Occurrence." *Journal of Health Communication* 13, no. 2 (2008): 107–124.

Zikmund-Fisher, B., et al. "Highlighting 'Additional Risk' Yields More Consistent Interpretations of Side Effect Risk Communications." *Medical Decision Making* 25, no. 1 (2005): E2.

Chapter 11: Coaching Patients to Be Partners

Besides the readings below, this chapter also draws on my interviews of Sherrie Kaplan and Jeff Belkora.

Anderson, L. A., et al. "Effects of Modeling on Patient Communication, Satisfaction, and Knowledge." *Medical Care* 25, no. 11 (1987): 1044–1056.

Greenfield, S., et al. "Patients' Participation in Medical Care: Effects on Blood Sugar Control and Quality of Life in Diabetes." *Journal of General Internal Medicine* 3, no. 5 (1988): 448–457.

Harrington, J., et al. "Improving Patients' Communication with Doctors: A Systematic Review of Intervention Studies." *Patient Education and Counseling* 52, no. 1 (2004): 7–16.

The Fifth Report of the Joint National Committee on Prevention, Detection, Evaluation, and Treatment of High Blood Pressure (JNC5). *Archives of Internal Medicine* 153, no. 2 (1993): 2413–2446.

Landro, L. "Weighty Choices, in Patients' Hands." *Wall Street Journal,* August 4, 2009. http://online.wsj.com/article/SB100014240529702036747045743285706 37446770.html

Langer, E. J., and J. Rodin. "The Effects of Choice and Enhanced Personal Responsibility for the Aged: A Field Experiment in an Institutional Setting." *Journal of Personality and Social Psychology* 34, no. 2 (1976): 191–198.

Robinson, E. J., and M. J. Whitfield. "Improving the Efficiency of Patients' Comprehension Monitoring: A Way of Increasing Patients' Participation in General Practice Consultations." *Social Science and Medicine* 21, no. 8 (1985): 915–919.

Rodin, J., and E. J. Langer. "Long-Term Effects of a Control-Relevant Intervention with the Institutionalized Aged." *Journal of Personality and Social Psychology* 35, no. 12 (1977): 897–902.

Chapter 12: The Limits of Patient Empowerment

Bartelink, H., et al. "Impact of a Higher Radiation Dose on Local Control and Survival in Breast-Conserving Therapy of Early Breast Cancer: 10-Year Results of the Randomized Boost Versus No Boost EORTC 22881–10882 Trial." *Journal of Clinical Oncology* 25, no. 22 (2007): 3259–3265.

Fellner, C. H., and J. R. Marshall. "Kidney Donors: The Myth of Informed Consent." *American Journal of Psychiatry* 126, no. 9 (1970): 1245–1251.

Kahneman, D. *Thinking, Fast and Slow.* New York: Farrar, Straus and Giroux, 2011.

Katz, S. J., et al. "Patient Involvement in Surgery Treatment Decisions for Breast Cancer." *Journal of Clinical Oncology* 23, no. 24 (2005): 5526–5533.

United States Preventive Services Task Force. "Screening for Breast Cancer: U.S. Preventive Services Task Force Recommendation Statement." *Annals of Internal Medicine* 151, no. 10 (2009): 716–726.

Weaver, D. L., et al. "Effect of Occult Metastases on Survival in Node-Negative Breast Cancer." *New England Journal of Medicine* 364, no. 5 (2011): 412–421.

Chapter 13: Preparing Physicians for Prepared Patients

For a more complete account of pizza and sex (and who wouldn't want a more complete account of those topics?), read Annie Janvier's amazing essay, cited below. This chapter also draws on personal communications with James Tulsky.

Ambady, N., et al. "Surgeon's Tone of Voice: A Clue to Malpractice History." *Surgery* 132, no. 1 (2002): 5–9.

Camerer, C., et al. "Neuroeconomics: How Neuroscience Can Inform Economics." *Journal of Economic Literature* 43, no. 1 (2005): 9–64.

Chua, H. F., et al. "Self-Related Neural Response to Tailored Smoking-Cessation Messages Predicts Quitting." *Natural Neuroscience* 14, no. 4 (2011): 426–427.

Eva, K. W., et al. "The Ability of the Multiple Mini-Interview to Predict Pre-Clerkship Performance in Medical School." *Academic Medicine* 79, no. 10 (2004): S40-S42.

Harris, G. "New for Aspiring Doctors, the People Skills Test." *New York Times*, July 11, 2011. New York edition p. A1.

Harris, S., and C. Owen. "Discerning Quality: Using the Multiple Mini-Interview in Student Selection for the Australian National University Medical School." *Medical Education* 41, no. 3 (2007): 234–241.

Inui, T. S., et al. "Improved Outcomes in Hypertension After Physician Tutorials." *Annals of Internal Medicine* 84, no. 6 (1976): 646–651.

Janvier, A. "Pepperoni Pizza and Sex." *Current Problems in Pediatric and Adolescent Health Care* 41, no. 4 (2011): 106–108.

Koropchak, C. M., et al. "Studying Communication in Oncologist–Patient Encounters: The SCOPE Trial." *Palliative Medicine* 20, no. 8 (2006): 813–819.

Kreiter, C. D., et al. "Investigating the Reliability of the Medical School Admissions Interview." *Advances in Health Sciences Education* 9, no. 2 (2004): 147–159.

Levinson, W., et al. "Physician–Patient Communication. The Relationship with Malpractice Claims Among Primary Care Physicians and Surgeons." *Journal of the American Medical Association* 277, no. 7 (1997): 553–559.

Localio, A. R., et al. "Relationship Between Malpractice Claims and Cesarean Delivery." *Journal of the American Medical Association* 269, no. 3 (1993): 366–373.

Reznick, R., et al. "An Objective Structured Clinical Examination for the Licentiate of the Medical Council of Canada: From Research to Reality." *Academic Medicine* 68, suppl. 10 (1993): S4–6.

Skinner, C. S., et al. "Use of and Reactions to a Tailored CD-ROM Designed to Enhance Oncologist–Patient Communication: The SCOPE Trial Intervention." *Patient Education and Counseling* 77, no. 1 (2009): 90–96.

White, J., et al. "Oh, by the Way . . ." *Journal of General Internal Medicine* 9, no. 1 (1994): 24–28.

Index

Scan this code with your smartphone to be linked to bonus materials for *CRITICAL DECISIONS* and other healthy living books and information.

You can also text keyword DECISIONS to READIT (732348) to be sent a link to the mobile website.